THE PHYTOZYME CURE

TREAT OR REVERSE MORE THAN
30 SERIOUS HEALTH CONDITIONS
WITH POWERFUL PLANT NUTRIENTS

MICHELLE SCHOFFRO COOK

BSc, RNCP, ROHP, DNM

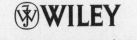

WILEY

John Wiley & Sons Canada, Ltd

Library and Archives Canada Cataloguing in Publication

Cook, Michelle Schoffro
   The phytozyme cure: treat or reverse more than 30 serious health conditions with powerful plant nutrients / Michelle Schoffro Cook.

Includes bibliographical references and index.
ISBN 978-0-470-15758-9

   1. Nutrition.   2. Functional foods.   3. Vegetables in human nutrition.
I. Title.

RM237.9.C66 2010   613.2'6   C2010-904377-4

Production Credits
Cover design: Diana Sullada
Cover photos: ©iStockphoto.com/Lenta (Bilberries)
     ©iStockphoto.com/PIKSEL (Hands full of cherries)
Interior design: Pat Loi
Typesetting: Thomson Digital
Printer: Friesens Printing

John Wiley & Sons Canada, Ltd.
6045 Freemont Blvd.
Mississauga, Ontario
L5R 4J3

Printed in Canada

1 2 3 4 5 FP 14 13 12 11 10

This book is dedicated to Curtis, the love of my life and my beautiful soul mate.

And to my wonderfully supportive parents, Michael and Deborah Schoffro.

Contents

Acknowledgments

I am fortunate to be surrounded by wonderful people of integrity who support me in my work and my personal life. I would like to thank all the kind and honest people who walk through life with me.

To my incredible husband and love, Curtis Cook, I am blessed to love and be loved by you. You are an incredible example of integrity, kindness, wisdom, and love. You are so much more than I ever dreamed possible and I am grateful to share life with you. Anyone who has been graced by knowing you knows that you are a wise soul who shines brilliantly. As this book goes to print, we celebrate our thirteenth beautiful year together. I loved you from the second I met you. With every passing day, my heart is more full of love because I know you. Thank you for your constant support, love, and wisdom. Your loving embrace heals me. Your love transforms me. Our souls are one. Always. Forever.

To my immensely supportive parents, Michael and Deborah Schoffro, thanks for your belief in me throughout my life. Thanks also for encouraging me to be a writer.

To my wonderful friend and expert medical reviewer, Carri Drzyzga, thanks for many years of friendship and support. Thanks also for sharing your brilliance.

To my agent, Claire Gerus, thanks for your assistance and support, particularly through the numerous difficulties that faced me during the writing of this book. Your valuable insights are always appreciated.

To everyone at Wiley who has contributed to this book, thank you for your assistance and for helping me to share this important information.

To Heather Ball, thank you for your fine editing of this book. You are a real professional and such a pleasure to work with.

To everyone who has supported me through friendship or in my work, thank you for helping me to fulfill my life's purpose.

Introduction

*We lift ourselves by our thought, we climb upon
our vision of ourselves. If you want to enlarge your
life, you must first enlarge your thought of it and of
yourself. Hold the ideal of yourself as you long to be,
always, everywhere—your ideal of what you long to
attain—the ideal of health, efficiency, success.*
—Orison Swett Marden

Destiny frequently has better plans for us than we might have ever considered. We may be so wrapped up in planning our own future that we may not appreciate the opportunities that lie before us. Perhaps that is because sometimes these opportunities are shrouded in pain and masked in hardship. Instead we may myopically see the crumbling plans and dashed dreams that we once held dear, potentially missing the calling or opportunity that awaits us. I know this firsthand. It is how I came to call natural medicine, holistic nutrition, and the healing arts my profession and passion . . . and my destiny.

In my late teens, I was diagnosed with a rare, incurable genetic disease. Little was (and still is) known about the condition, and few treatment options exist or existed. But despite my health problems, I was determined to live out what I clearly perceived as my destiny: a career as an international journalist, stationed in war-torn nations, relaying the stories of people worldwide. But destiny had other plans for me.

Partway through journalism school, a physician who was monitoring my health decided to change my treatment plan and switched my medication; a decision that would have dire consequences for me. Within days, I was largely confined to bed. At the worst of times I was unable to move; at the best of times I could walk only a few steps. While I switched back to the original medication, the damage had been done. Unable to get out of bed on most days, I had to withdraw from journalism school to regain my health.

My nineteenth birthday came and went without fanfare. I lay bedridden, as months, then years, passed. I felt as though I was drowning in a million tears, paralyzed by exhaustion and weakness. The words of my physician, specialist of specialists and the twentieth or so whom I had consulted, echoed in my head: "There is no cure. The disease will only get worse. You will need medication for the rest of your life just to keep you alive. You will certainly die without it. There is nothing else we can do for you."

On the rare occasions when I could lift my limbs to leave the bed, I sought refuge by sitting in the sun. The warmth of its rays and the fresh smell of the outdoor air gave me a sense of peace and took my mind off my problems. This was my first clue that perhaps nature offered me healing where the medical system had failed.

In the moments when I could sit up and read, I began to study nutrition by distance education. As I began to practice some of the dietary suggestions I was learning about, I started to notice changes in my health: I had more energy, better movement, and increased healing.

Slowly I began to feel better, and I immersed myself more fully into my studies of natural medicine and nutrition. When I could, I even ventured out into a nearby forest and picked plants that I dried or preserved to use as remedies.

As my healing progressed further, I started working part time at a local natural food store, sharing my knowledge with people seeking to regain their health after the medical system had failed them, too. Eventually, I was able to start my own health food store and nutritional consulting practice. Finally I was on my path, I thought.

But destiny interrupted my plans again. A horrendous car accident left me bedridden, this time with excruciating pain from migraines, fractured bones, scar tissue, fibromyalgia, partial paralysis from a spinal cord injury, and permanent breathing impairment from a brain injury. I wondered how the universe could leave me in this state after I had worked so tirelessly to regain my health. Being only 21 by this time, I refused to accept that this was to be my life. So, I continued to use my body as my laboratory, testing foods, herbs, healing remedies, and therapies. Month after month and year after year, my health continued to improve.

When the light of my life and dreams seemed snuffed out so violently, the universe was actually sharing some of its most miraculous teachings, leading me to the natural medicines that offer so much more than pharmaceutical drugs, and the natural remedies and therapies that give so much more hope than surgery. While I had other plans for my life, destiny, too, had its own plans for me. What once seemed a curse became a tremendous blessing.

Today, while I have not completely cured the genetic disease, I have dramatically reduced the pain my body experiences, I have much more energy than I used to, and I have lived for 16 years completely free of the medication that once kept me alive—16 years longer than the medical profession had given me. I still have occasional setbacks, but I have survived, and even thrived, in the face of great odds. And, as I continue to use the natural approaches of the Phytozyme Cure, I experience greater health.

Many years passed and I consulted with many beautiful people suffering from tragic health circumstances. I poured my heart into helping them, continuing my research to find solutions to assist them in their recovery. I witnessed miracles. Client after client shared his or her healing experiences as we employed the research and natural remedies I was drawn to use. Words cannot impart the humbling experience of playing a role in another's healing. I knew that more people needed this information than I could reach on a one-on-one basis.

Now, I see that destiny wanted me to share with you the wisdom of nature in the form of this book, *The Phytozyme Cure*. For me, there is no nobler use for the pen (or computer, as is the case now) than to help others have a better quality of life, and perhaps to live a longer, better life than they might have otherwise. And, when I discovered the healing power of phytonutrients and enzymes, which I call Phytozyme Therapy, I wanted everyone to know about their abilities to heal and improve health.

I believe that phytonutrients (also called micronutrients) and enzymes will play a significant role in the future of medicine, but right now most people haven't even heard of them, or if they have, they are misinformed. You might have heard that enzymes support only the digestive process. It's true that some enzymes can improve digestion, but that's only the beginning. These molecular power-houses not only heal but in some cases they even reverse illness.

In *The Phytozyme Cure*, I explain that enzyme deficiencies are factors in many health problems. Without adequate enzymes, we are unable to digest the foods (including nutritional supplements) we eat or absorb the nutrients they contain. Without these building blocks of healthy cells and organs, we often suffer severe health consequences.

The important information in this book will help you experience greater energy and vitality, prevent illness, and reverse disease. *The Phytozyme Cure* is packed with information on phytonutrients and enzymes and reveals their amazing functions in our bodies.

The Phytozyme Cure guides you to maximize the curative properties of phytonutrients and enzymes for optimal healing. It is backed by the most cutting-edge research on phytonutrients and enzyme therapy—a field virtually untouched in today's drug-based medicine—and includes the latest scientific findings about the power of these natural substances.

Science has revealed that phytonutrients can speed weight loss in people who are overweight, prevent heart disease and cancer, and even reverse some of the effects of aging and brain damage. Research has also shown the roles specific enzymes play in attacking cancer cells in the body and removing toxins linked to such conditions as nerve pain and facial paralysis. There is also evidence that other enzymes can break down infectious bacteria and viruses, or remove dead or scar tissue resulting from injuries, burns, or wounds. And the newest research shows that enzymes can even help the body grow healthy new tissue, skin, and hair.

But the greatest health benefits can be realized when these two powerhouses (phytonutrients and enzymes) work together. Phytozyme Therapy is an exciting new natural approach to healing. It is a powerful diet- and nutrition-based therapy I developed based on two decades of research and clinical experience. It involves a multifaceted approach to health and wellness:

1. *Determining your specific enzyme weaknesses.* Everyone has biochemical strengths and weaknesses; however, it is our weaknesses that determine whether we will experience health issues and, if so, which ones. Determining your biochemical weakness can empower you to make simple but critical dietary modifications that are specific to your body's needs so you can potentially prevent illness from forming or to help your body heal from illness if it has already settled in.

2. *Adding specific phytonutrient-rich foods, phytonutrient supplements, and other natural remedies.* Doing so will dramatically bolster your body's healing abilities.

3. *Using specific enzymes to remove the barriers to health.* These barriers might include inflammation, pathogens (viruses, bacteria, fungi, and other microbes), or cancer cells. Research supports supplementing with enzymes to treat these issues.

The combination of addressing one's metabolic weaknesses, adding substances to speed and improve healing, and removing the barriers to healing work together to dramatically improve your health. And, there are added benefits to Phytozyme Therapy:

- **Faster healing**.
- **Improved energy**.
- **Greater mental clarity**.
- **Increased resistance to illness**.
- **Financial savings**. Many people take supplements in an ad hoc fashion with no clear plan, which can be an expensive waste of time. *The Phytozyme Cure* will guide you to the best choices for your specific health condition, resulting in savings in your pockets and a lighter load for your digestive tract and liver.
- **Healing of serious health conditions.** As I researched possible cures and healing methods for me and my clients, I discovered that many illnesses—even serious ones—can be improved or reversed using the specific combinations of phytonutrients and enzymes that I share here. What's more, these powerful healing substances are completely natural, and many can be found in common foods like fruits and vegetables.

In my one-on-one natural medicine and nutritional consultations with clients, I have seen people healed of all kinds of illnesses. One woman had relentless back pain for six years. Within months of her treatment with Phytozyme Therapy, she was pain-free and motorcycling across the countryside. Another woman had suffered from fibromyalgia for over a decade. In a matter of months, she was symptom-free and entering cycling competitions. I have seen children with learning disabilities make dramatic improvements, and have witnessed significant healing in men and women suffering from allergies, infections, and even cancer—and frequently saw their illnesses reverse altogether. Even I was surprised by the tremendous results.

Now, I'm not suggesting that Phytozyme Therapy is a cure-all. It isn't. But it works marvelously in many cases. I've included protocols to address over 30 health conditions in Part Two of this book, and if you suffer from one or more of these conditions, I believe Phytozyme Therapy can help you. While most people will find their health issues covered among these protocols, the Phytozyme Cure still works on many other health conditions. So don't be disappointed if you don't see your condition listed—the Phytozyme Cure still holds tremendous promise for you.

The problem with many nutrition and diet plans is that they offer a one-size-fits-all approach. Time and again, my clients describe trying countless new supplements and diets, only to be discouraged because nothing worked. But what makes the Phytozyme Cure so beneficial is that I've created a reliable, strategic, and individualized approach. Through the Phytozyme Cure, we can arm our bodies with the tools to overcome disease and enjoy long-term healthy living. I strove to create a reliable, strategic, and *individualized* approach that anyone can use: the average person who wants to manage his or her own health; the natural health practitioner who wants to get better results in his or her practice; or the medical clinician who wants to dramatically affect healing, not just eliminate the symptoms of an illness. And that is just what Phytozyme Therapy delivers.

With the Phytozyme Cure, you can overcome your particular biochemical weaknesses (we all have them) and experience optimal health. You'll learn the specific foods, dietary suggestions, and supplement guidelines for your specific health needs so you can start benefiting from this powerful knowledge immediately.

I help you discover what you need to maximize your healing potential, prevent illness and disease, and achieve better health. Then, fueled by optimum foods and supplements, you'll finally experience the abundant energy, renewed youthful appearance, and supercharged immune system you deserve.

The Phytozyme Cure provides a clear program that you can follow. You don't need to be a biochemist specializing in phytonutrients or an enzymologist to start benefiting from Phytozyme Therapy today, because this book takes the guesswork out of selecting the right enzyme supplements for your body. You will learn how to choose the right enzyme supplements to support digestion, relieve pain, maximize healing, and even reverse many common health concerns.

Close to two decades of scientific research, as well as clinical and personal experience, have led me to the conclusion that nature and natural medicines hold the secret to health and healing. But I never would have discovered these amazing healing substances had I not had some unfortunate health experiences and then been open to the new roads destiny was trying to show me. It is my hope that through the Phytozyme Cure you will embrace a new destiny for yourself, one of a longer, healthier, and happier life.

PART**ONE**

Combining Phytonutrients and Enzymes for Optimum Health and Healing

1

Phyto Power in the Fight Against Disease

Each one of the substances of a man's diet acts upon
his body and changes it in some way, and upon these
changes, his whole life depends, whether he be in
health, in sickness, or convalescent.

—Hippocrates

During the Age of Exploration, much of the world was largely unknown to Europeans, and the Americas that are now home to millions of people were completely unknown except to the aboriginal people who inhabited them. As our history books tell us, Christopher Columbus set sail to find a passage to India that would help him access Asian spices, which were traded like currency at the time. Battling harsh seas, and possibly homesickness, was not all that confronted Columbus during his months-long voyages. Perhaps his greatest challenge was sickness among his crew. Many of the men on the *Santa Maria* suffered from swollen and bleeding gums, sore joints, bleeding under the skin, bruises and blemishes on the legs, and wounds that did not heal. Some eventually died from the disease, which has since become known as scurvy.

Legend has it that some of the Portuguese men suffering from scurvy asked to be released onto what they believed was a deserted island, where they could die in peace, rather than face death on the ship. According to this legend, the men ate fruit and greens they found on the island, now known as Curaçao and, thanks to the produce's vitamin C content, their scurvy was cured. (Incidentally, "curaçao" derives from the Portuguese word for "to cure"—reflective of the cure that awaited these early settlers.)

We now know that without vitamin C humans will inevitably suffer from scurvy. Over the years scientists discovered that deficiencies in vitamins B1 (thiamine), B3 (niacin), and D are also linked to diseases: beriberi, pellagra, and rickets respectively. And, by their very definition, vitamins are nutrients that are essential to maintain our health.

Nutrition to Prevent and Treat Disease

Although we've explored most corners of world geography, when it comes to nutrition, we're still in an age of exploration. Over the years, scientists have discovered many more vitamins and dozens of minerals that are essential to warding off specific diseases. Micronutrients, as vitamins and minerals are also called, are essential for the health of our cells, tissues, and organs, and, therefore, to our overall health as well. Our understanding of these essential nutrients has skyrocketed over the last few decades, and we now know much more about the role they play in helping us to grow healthy bones, brains, glands, and organs. (To learn more about these vital nutrients and their roles in supporting a healthy body, consult my book *The Life Force Diet*.)

Our understanding of nutrition to prevent or treat disease has now gone well beyond the role of vitamins and minerals, and we know more than ever about how the foods we eat (or don't eat) determine the state of our health. Scientific advances have proven that, for example, we need essential fatty acids (like omega-3s) for proper brain development and health; we need adequate magnesium to ward off depression and for healthy nerve transmission; and we need vitamin D for strong bones, balanced moods, and the ability to fight off viruses.

But that understanding of nutrition and its role in creating healthy cells, tissues, organs, and organ systems is just the tip of the iceberg, and current nutrition research is moving in many exciting directions.

One direction includes the scientific research into the role nutrition plays in not just avoiding nutritional deficiency diseases but in preventing *genetic* diseases, which were once thought inevitable, from developing. This field of research, nutrigenomics, is the study of genetic responses to nutrition as well as the role of nutrition to support genetic well-being. It holds substantial promise in the discovery of natural solutions for preventing and possibly even reversing serious illness, genetic diseases included.

Over the last decade we've learned that nutrients, or the lack of them, can determine whether our genes will mutate to cause disease or whether they'll keep us healthy and immune to it—even to genetic diseases to which we are predisposed. That's mind boggling if you think about it!

Now that scientists have stacks of research on macronutrients— like amino acids from protein foods, essential fatty acids from fatty foods, and sugars from carbohydrates—many have turned their attention to micronutrients. And most recently, science has begun to unlock the door to a realm of nutrients we've only just begun to explore: phytonutrients and enzymes.

Exploring Phytonutrients

You may have heard of phytonutrients, or phytochemicals or nutra-ceuticals, as they are also called. But even if you haven't, I'm sure you've experienced them. Every time you drink a cup of coffee and feel the adrenalin rush and the resulting energy burst that caffeine provides, you've experienced the effects of phytonutrients. In this case, caffeine is the phytonutrient that bolstered your energy. Every time you eat an orange, the brilliant orange color, appetizing scent, and delicious taste are all the result of phytonutrients. But they don't just impart color, scent, and taste; phytonutrients assist with burning fat and warding off cancer, diabetes, and stroke, among other conditions.

So what exactly is a phytonutrient or phytochemical? "Phyto" is derived from the Greek word "phyton," which means plant. So, phytonutrients are plant-based micronutrients. But because scientists could not determine any symptoms of phytonutrient deficiencies in people (unlike vitamin deficiencies), phytonutrients are not technically considered necessary for health and proper body function. But that doesn't mean they aren't important.

Fast Facts: Phytonutrients

Phytonutrients are the active health-protecting, nonessential compounds that are found in plants like fruits, vegetables, herbs, spices, nuts, sprouts, and seeds. Phytonutrients give plant foods their color, aroma, taste, and immune system. A single fruit or vegetable may contain more than one hundred types of healing phytonutrients. For example, spinach contains beta-carotene, lutein, zeaxanthin, alpha lipoic acid, chlorophyll, and more. Eating phytonutrients can enhance immunity, fight cancer, protect genes, and provide many other health benefits.

As science is discovering, phytonutrients are potent substances that have the power to prevent and, in some cases, treat many diseases. There are currently about five thousand known kinds, and scientists are discovering new phytonutrients and their many healing properties almost daily. Once you know more about their health marvels, I'm sure you'll want them in your diet.

The Benefits of Phytonutrients

When you eat phytonutrients, they impart their potent healing abilities inside your body. Some have antioxidant properties—meaning that they destroy free radicals in your body that are linked to most diseases and aging. Others help balance hormones or protect your eyes against damage and degeneration. Still others have antibacterial, antifungal, or antiviral properties. Some even prevent damage to blood vessels linked to heart disease, while others help protect your body's genetic material against damage.

Other specific phytonutrients even have anticancer properties, which can help your body fight cancer by

1. slowing the reproduction of cancer cells,
2. causing cancer cells to commit suicide (called apoptosis),
3. preventing the growth of new blood vessels that nourish cancer tumors,
4. preventing substances in the body from being converted to carcinogens, and
5. encouraging enzymes that link to carcinogens and then remove them from the body.

Don't let their rainbow colors and aromatic scents fool you: phytonutrients mean business. Combined with enzymes (I tell you more about enzymes in Chapter 2), they can help you experience boundless energy, disease-free living, and even slow the aging process.

Three Great Groups of Phytonutrients

The thousands of phytonutrients are categorized into major groups, some of which include carotenoids, phenolics, sterols, and terpenes. Each of the categories is further subdivided into specific phytonutrients or phytonutrient subgroups. Don't worry, you don't have to memorize their names or classifications, know their chemical structure, or even be able to pronounce them to benefit from their healing properties.[1] While there are many different phytonutrient classifications, here's an overview of three of the most healing ones: carotenoids, flavonoids, and sterols.

Carotenoids—Adding Color and Health

Carotenoids are a group of phytonutrients that provide the yellow-orange-red pigments found in foods like carrots, sweet potatoes, apricots, mangoes, pumpkin, tomatoes, papaya, peaches, squash, and other similarly colored foods. You may have heard of beta-carotene, lutein, and lycopene, all of which are specific types of carotenoids. While there are over 700 different carotenoids in nature, only about 60 are found in food.[2] And the average person in North America eats fewer than a dozen different kinds and only in modest amounts. Some carotenoids, specifically alpha-carotene, beta-carotene, and cryptoxanthin, convert to vitamin A in our bodies, which is essential for healthy skin and vision. While carotenoids' ability to form vitamin A is important, they play other valuable roles.

Not only do carotenoids help strengthen our eyesight and boost our immunity to disease, they are powerful antioxidants that help ward off cancer and protect against the effects of aging. Studies at Harvard University of more than 124,000 people showed a 32 percent reduction in risk of lung cancer in people who consumed a variety of carotenoid-rich foods as part of their regular diet.[3] Women's Healthy Eating and Living (WHEL) conducted a study of women who had completed treatment for early-stage breast cancer. Researchers found that women with the highest blood concentrations of carotenoids had the least likelihood of cancer recurrence.[4]

Besides the brilliantly colored foods I mentioned earlier, dark green vegetables like broccoli, and leafy greens like collard, kale, and spinach also contain high amounts of carotenoids.

Flavonoids—Nature's Potent Anti-Inflammatories

Found in nuts, berries, and tea, phenolics (or phenols or polyphenols, as they are sometimes called) are powerful antioxidants with anti-inflammatory properties. In addition, they are antiallergenic, meaning that they help reduce the biochemical processes that cause allergic reactions. You may have read about flavonoids—one group of phenolics that is showing huge promise against many illnesses and in the prevention of disease. Flavonoids interfere with the development of cancer cells and prevent them from multiplying. They include anthocyanins, catechins, hesperetin, isoflavones, naringin, quercetin, rutin, silymarin, tangeretin, and tannins.

Foods such as berries, cherries, currants, pomegranates, red and purple grapes, red onions, tomatoes, bell peppers, apples, tea, and walnuts contain flavonoids.

Sterols—Healing Hormones

Sterols are phytonutrients that are essentially plant hormones. One in particular, beta-sitosterol, is basically plant cholesterol. You may be surprised to learn that this plant cholesterol has powerful healing abilities when ingested and can actually be helpful to reduce harmful LDL cholesterol in humans.

The A to Z of Healing with Phytonutrients

Now, let's further explore the many health rewards of phytonutrients. For the purposes of *The Phytozyme Cure,* we'll be focusing on 31 main kinds, but I promise you don't need a chemistry degree to follow along. Here, I show you the powerful medicinal properties phytochemicals and the foods that contain them, so you can easily incorporate them into your diet.

Alpha-Carotene

A study of six types of carotenoids in relation to the risk of developing cancer found that low levels of four of the carotenoids were linked to a higher incidence of lung cancer. Specifically, researchers found that low levels of alpha-carotene, beta-carotene, cryptoxanthin, and lycopene correlate to a high incidence of lung cancer. This was particularly true of alpha-carotene.[5]

Anthocyanins

These natural, health-boosting substances give certain fruits their purple to reddish color. Not only does research show that anthocyanins have the capacity to boost short-term memory by 100 percent in just eight weeks, they also stimulate the burning of stored fat in the body to be used as fuel. Research published in the *Journal of Agricultural and Food Chemistry* found that a group of laboratory animals which ate a high-fat diet along with anthocyanins gained 24 percent less weight than their counterparts which ate only a fatty diet.[6] Anthocyanins are found in berries, cherries, and dark purple and red grapes.

Astaxanthin

Astaxanthin is nature's protection against ultraviolet (UV) rays. It helps prevent sun damage to skin, improves skin elasticity, and may reduce wrinkling. Research indicates that it may increase cellular energy, protect against cancer, protect against damage to the brain and nervous system, and slow diabetes-related health complications.[7] Other research indicates that it ameliorates genetic damage and may protect against free radical damage to the liver, as well as liver and colon cancer.[8] Because astaxanthin is such a potent antioxidant, it is also showing promise for arthritis and other pain disorders, as well as heart disease.[9] It is found in carrots, red peppers, and red-colored fruits and vegetables.

Beta-Carotene

Like alpha-carotene, beta-carotene is a powerful antioxidant that converts to vitamin A in the body. It is the most abundant carotenoid in our diet and has been the subject of scientific scrutiny, thanks to a controversial study that is interestingly called the CARET study.

The CARET study tested a low dose of beta-carotene and/or 25,000 IU (international units) of vitamin A on men and women at a high risk of developing lung cancer. The subjects had either been exposed to asbestos and/or were heavy smokers. In the study, those people taking beta-carotene with vitamin A had a 28 percent higher rate of mortality from lung cancer and a 17 percent increase in mortality compared to the placebo group. Of course, the media became a bit crazed about these findings and, without exploring the possibility of flaws in the study, informed people that beta-carotene contributes to disease, which of course, is not true. For example, the *Seattle Times* and the *Los Angeles Times* featured a story declaring: "Beta Carotene May Cause, Not Prevent, Cancer."[10]

I, like many nutritionists, believe that the CARET study may have been flawed for a number of reasons:

1. As Lester Packer, PhD, director of the Packer Lab at the University of California at Berkeley, so aptly stated, "The participants in the CARET study were walking time bombs ... It may simply have been too late to make a difference for this group" and they may not have been the best subjects for such a study.[11]
2. Not all beta-carotenes are created equally. The researchers used a synthetic version that is not identical to beta-carotene found in food—the form that is best used by the body.
3. The participants used beta-carotene on its own, when research demonstrates that the carotenoids work best as a team—in other words, combined with other carotenoids.
4. The supplementation may have accelerated existing cancers. If you're a heavy drinker or smoker, or have been exposed to asbestos, it is probably best that you stay clear of beta-carotene supplementation.

Since that unfortunate study, there have been other well-conceived ones that espouse the benefits of beta-carotene. Dr. Michelle Santos of the USDA Human Nutrition Center on Aging found that supplementation of 50 milligrams of beta-carotene resulted in stronger immune system activity in the 65- to 85-year-old men she studied. Actually, she found that their immune systems returned to levels comparable to men 20 years their junior.[12]

Beta-Sitosterol

Beta-sitosterol is the plant version of cholesterol but, ironically, it appears to lower cholesterol levels in humans by blocking the absorption of cholesterol. Research shows that beta-sitosterol has a beneficial effect on men with prostate enlargement. Because it is an antioxidant it lessens free radical damage to the body and appears to offer protection against some forms of cancer, including breast, colon, and prostate cancer. In research, beta-sitosterol encouraged cancer cells to commit suicide, lessened their ability to proliferate, and in breast cancer, sought out and destroyed cancer cells while leaving healthy cells unscathed.[13] This important phytonutrient is primarily found in corn oil, flaxseed, peanuts, pumpkin seeds, rice bran, soybeans, and wheat germ. Choose only organic corn oil and soybeans, since non-organic versions of these crops are heavily genetically modified.

Capsaicin

This phytonutrient turns up the heat! If you've ever eaten spicy food, chances are that you are familiar with the work of this powerful healing substance. Found in chilies, capsaicin is a powerful healing phytonutrient. It is an anti-inflammatory that can dramatically reduce pain and is used in many topical pain creams. Capsaicin interacts with nerve cells, sending signals back to the brain to reduce or stop the pain cycle, and consuming capsaicin causes your body to release feel-good hormones called endorphins. According to research, capsaicin can effectively relieve arthritic symptoms and improve joint flexibility. It may also protect against gastric ulcers by increasing blood flow to the membrane of the stomach. Plus, research shows that capsaicin-based creams or ointments reduce the itching, scaling, and redness of psoriasis.[14]

Catechins

The full name for these natural plant compounds is catechin polyphenols. They activate fat-burning genes in abdominal fat cells to assist with weight loss, and belly fat loss in particular. According to research at Tufts University, catechins increase abdominal fat loss by 77 percent and double total weight loss. As if that wasn't enough reason for most of us to include foods high in catechins, like green and black tea, in our diets, catechins also improve your body's ability to use insulin secreted by your pancreas, which prevents blood sugar spikes and crashes involved in plummeting energy levels, cravings, depression, and mood swings.

Scientists have even discovered that epigallocatechin gallate (or EGCG for short), a particular type of catechin, is two hundred times more powerful at eliminating free radicals that damage the skin than vitamin E.[15]

Chlorogenic Acid

In early studies, chlorogenic acid has shown promise against cancer, particularly against liver cancer. It may also be helpful for weight loss and diabetes. Chlorogenic acid is primarily found in apples, carrots, coffee, flaxseed, pineapple, potatoes, and strawberries.

Cryptoxanthin

This carotenoid has shown promise in protecting women against cervical cancer. A study found that women who consumed higher levels of cryptoxanthin had significantly lower rates of cervical cancer than those who consumed less.[16] You can take advantage of its benefits by eating oranges, papayas, peaches, and tangerines.

Curcumin

Turmeric *(Curcuma longa)* is a yellowish spice commonly used in Indian food. Its main therapeutic ingredient is curcumin, which is a potent antioxidant and anti-inflammatory agent. It has been shown to play a role in pain disorders and brain disease. Research shows that curcumin suppresses pain by acting in a similar way to the class of drugs known as COX-2 inhibitors (without the harmful side effects), making it effective for pain.

Early evidence of the link between inflammation and Alzheimer's disease started when researchers Patrick McGeer at the University of British Columbia and Joe Rogers of Sun Health Research Institute in Arizona sifted through a decade of hospital drug records. They found that arthritis patients who were regularly treated with strong anti-inflammatories were seven times less likely to develop Alzheimer's.[17] Seven times! Since then, researchers have been looking for effective natural medicines against inflammation, and that is where curcumin really shines.

Recent findings indicate that ingesting 1200 milligrams of curcumin, the main therapeutic constituent of the spice turmeric, had the same effect as taking 300 milligrams of the anti-inflammatory drug phenylbutazone.[18]

Ellagic Acid

Ellagic acid shows anticancer and genetic material-protection capabilities. It encourages a healthy rate of apoptosis—how the body seeks out and destroys harmful or damaged cells, like cancer cells. Ellagic acid helps stimulate your liver's detoxification enzymes, so your liver can eliminate environmental toxins, excess hormones, and food toxins, and perform its hundreds of important functions normally.

Because whiskey contains ellagic acid, some people jokingly claim whiskey is a health food, which is a bit of a stretch. It is far better to obtain ellagic acid from blackberries, blueberries, sweet and sour cherries, black and red currants, elderberries, grapes, raspberries, and strawberries, than to drink alcohol, which is a neurotoxin (damages brain and nervous system cells) and hormone-disruptor.

Ferulic Acid

Ferulic acid is a strong antioxidant. It protects against skin damage from UV rays and damage to our genetic material. It lowers blood sugar levels and may be helpful for diabetes.[19] Research published in the journal *Carcinogenesis* showed that ferulic acid may help protect against cancer as well.[20]

Wheat bran is a good source of ferulic acid. Like its cousin ellagic acid, ferulic acid is also found in blackberries, blueberries, sweet and sour cherries, black and red currants, elderberries, grapes, raspberries, and strawberries.

Hesperetin/Hesperidin

Hesperetin and hesperidin are almost identical except that the latter is bound to a sugar molecule. Research shows that these potent phytonutrients have antioxidant, anti-inflammatory, anticarcinogenic, and cholesterol-lowering actions, and also protect blood vessels against damage. Hesperidin can also be beneficial for treating allergies and hay fever because it has antihistamine properties.[21]

A study published in the *Journal of Nutrition* found that hesperidin not only lowered cholesterol in the liver and blood of mice, it inhibited bone loss as well. While the research on the latter health application is still in its infancy, this could mean that hesperidin may help to prevent and treat osteoporosis.[22]

Green vegetables are a source of hesperidin/hesperetin, and you can find them in their highest concentration in citrus fruits like lemons and oranges, especially the white part, or pith.

Indole-3-Carbinol (I3C)

Indole-3-carbinol has shown tremendous promise against cancer by working on five levels:[23]

1. It protects against carcinogenic toxins.
2. It induces enzymes that metabolize carcinogens.
3. It helps repair genetic material.
4. It causes cancer cells to commit suicide (apoptosis).
5. It blocks estrogen receptor sites to protect against estrogen-dependent cancers like breast and cervical.

It is found primarily in cruciferous vegetables, including broccoli, broccoli sprouts, brussels sprouts, cabbage, cauliflower, and kale.

Isoflavones

Isoflavones are the most common type of phytoestrogens, which are natural plant hormones. They play an important role in helping to regulate hormones in humans, to reduce our chances of developing hormone-related cancers like breast and prostate cancer, as well as assisting with maintaining a healthy hormone balance during peri-menopause and menopause. Phytoestrogens are naturally found in seeds, grains, some fruits and vegetables, and in higher quantities in soy foods like soy milk and tofu.

A lot of misinformation regarding isoflavones is out there, due to their ability to function like estrogen in our bodies. Many health practitioners are even misguided about isoflavones. Let me try to set the record straight.

Genistein is the phytoestrogen that is the most like estrogen of all the isoflavones, and it can actually balance out our bodies' estrogen levels. That's because when our bodies have too much estrogen and we ingest weak plant estrogens in the form of genistein, these can bind to the receptors and stop our bodies from producing more estrogen, or prevent our bodies' own estrogen from binding to these sites. Because plant estrogens are weaker, they can help lower our estrogen levels. Conversely, if we do not have enough estrogen, ingesting more through foods helps to increase the amount of estrogen in our bodies.

Genistein has many other health benefits, including being an antioxidant, having anticancer properties, and even helping with metabolic syndrome. It is also helpful in preventing heart attacks and strokes, since it acts as an anticlotting agent.[24] While many doctors tell people to avoid genistein if they are at risk for hormone-related cancers (particularly breast and prostate cancer), research shows that consuming isoflavones like genistein may actually protect against these forms of cancer.[25] Many doctors wrongly assume that because estrogen can make hormone-related cancers worse, taking phytoestrogen will do the same. But this isoflavone can actually be helpful, because it binds to estrogen receptors, which reduce your body's own manufacture of estrogen or its ability to bind to the receptors and initiate cancer growth.

You can find genistein primarily in soybeans and soy foods like miso, tempeh, tofu, and in small amounts in chickpeas (garbanzo beans).

Lipoic Acid

Lipoic acid is a powerful antioxidant that has the ability to mop up free radicals linked to aging and disease. In addition, within cells, it can increase the production of leptin, which appears to stifle the production of the chemical ghrelin, which is linked to increased appetite. In other words, lipoic acid can help turn off hunger pangs! Overweight women taking lipoic acid in scientific studies were found to have lost 5 percent of their body weight within six months.[26] Lipoic acid has also been shown to power up the energy centers of the cells, called mitochondria, helping them to work more effectively—that means more energy for you! Researchers at the University of California at Berkeley found that supplementation with lipoic acid doubled energy levels in their subjects.

Lipoic acid is found in plentiful amounts in dark leafy greens, including collard greens, kale, spinach, and Swiss chard.

Lutein

Like its cousins in the carotenoid family, lutein is an antioxidant. Research shows that it may prevent the hardening and narrowing of arteries linked to heart disease. And because it might also lower the risk of age-related vision loss,[27] people use lutein extensively as a natural treatment for macular degeneration. In a study called The Physicians' Health Study, conducted by Harvard scientists, researchers found that lower levels of lutein (as well as other carotenoids) are linked to increased risk of stroke.[28]

Avocadoes are rich sources of lutein.

Lycopene

Lycopene is considered to be the most potent antioxidant of all the carotenoids. It has a strong protective effect against pancreatic cancer.[29] According to research, it may also protect against prostate cancer, atherosclerosis, and asthma.[30] Studies show that it may help protect against other forms of cancer as well.[31] There is early research to suggest that it may help protect against hypertension and cardiovascular disease, osteoporosis, and nervous system disorders.[32] The higher the levels of lycopene in a person's blood and tissues, the lower his or her risk of cancer, particularly prostate and breast, as research shows.[33] It may even help protect against radiation.[34]

While the heat from cooking destroys most nutrients, lycopene appears to withstand heat, and cooking it actually increases its absorbability by the body. So tomato sauce is an excellent choice for getting lycopene in your diet, because it is found in tomatoes. You can also get lycopene from pink grapefruit, guavas, papayas, rose hips, strawberries, and watermelon.

Naringin

Naringin is the bitter-tasting compound in grapefruit. It has antioxidant and anticancer effects. Research shows that not only do grapefruit and naringin help prevent high cholesterol, they help lower cholesterol levels if they are already high.[35] Naringin also helps fight retinal disease in diabetics.[36] In rat studies, naringin showed a protective effect against brain injury linked to lack of oxygen—the type common with stroke.[37]

Perrillyl Alcohol

Early research on perrillyl alcohol suggests that it may have anticancer potential, namely because it appears to slow cancerous cell division and increase suicide rates of cancer cells.[38] Cherries and mint are good sources of this phytonutrient compound.

Proanthocyanidins

You may have heard that red wine has many health benefits. That's because it contains proanthocyanidins, which are potent antioxidant chemicals. They are powerful destroyers of free radicals, and may even protect against the effects of tobacco smoke and pollution. Proanthocyanidins show the unique ability to protect the brain from some environmental toxins, because they decrease free radical activity in and between brain cells.[39]

This phytonutrient may also offer good news to allergy sufferers. In research, proanthocyanidins inhibit the production of histamine, making them a natural anti-histamine without the drowsy side effect of many pharmaceuticals. Numerous studies show that proantho-cyanidins have anticancer and antitumor activity, and one study concluded that proanthocyanidins may demonstrate chemothera-peutic activity against breast cancer.

When it comes to heart disease, proanthocyanidins help reduce high blood pressure and improve the body's ability to metabolize fat. In tests on rabbits, proanthocyanidins demonstrated significant reduction in the development of atherosclerosis. They also appeared to protect against heart attacks linked to certain asthma drugs.[40] Research shows that proanthocyanidins have greater antioxidant properties than either vitamins C or E.

Proanthocyanidins are primarily found in dark red- to purple-colored fruits like blueberries, cherries, cranberries, grapes, raspberries, and strawberries, as well as in almonds, apples, cocoa, and peanuts.

Quercetin

This phytonutrient is best known for inhibiting the release of histamine—the chemical responsible for the uncomfortable symptoms of seasonal allergies. Quercetin has antioxidant and anti-inflammatory effects as well. Studies have found that eating a quercetin-rich diet lowers LDL (harmful) cholesterol, blood pressure, and risk of heart disease, as well as the risk of prostate, colon, ovarian, breast, gastric, prostate, and cervical cancers.[41]

Apples are an excellent source of quercetin, and some studies show that people who eat a lot of apples have improved lung function and reduced risk of lung diseases. While not certain, this protective quality may be linked to the quercetin in apples.

In addition to apples, you can find quercetin in berries, cabbage, cauliflower, nuts, onions, and black, green, or white tea.

Resveratrol

The flavonoid resveratrol has been getting a tremendous amount of media exposure due to its powerful ability to protect the brain from damage. Dr. Egemen Savaskan and colleagues at the University of Basel in Switzerland discovered resveratrol in grapes, which are currently the best-known source of this potent healing substance. They found that resveratrol mops up free radicals and protected brain cells from plaque that is linked to Alzheimer's.

Resveratrol offers many other health benefits. As well as being a powerful antioxidant, it may protect against damage caused by high blood sugar in diabetics; protect the heart and blood vessels against heart disease; and have antitoxic effects that support the liver and brain. Resveratrol helps protect against cancer by inhibiting the growth of cancer cells and protecting DNA from damage.[42] It is found in purple grapes, purple grape juice, red wine, and to a lesser extent in raspberries and blueberries.

Rutin

Like other flavonoids, rutin is essential for absorbing vitamin C. Rutin improves eye health, strengthens blood vessels—especially capillaries—reduces cholesterol levels, improves blood circulation, and acts as an antioxidant against free radical damage. Because it can strengthen eyes and capillaries, it is particularly helpful for diabetic retinopathy.

Get more rutin in your diet from citrus fruits, red apples, apricots, blackberries, broccoli, buckwheat, cherries, black currants, grapes, nuts, onions, peppers, plums, prunes, rose hips, tea, and bilberry fruit.

Saponins

Saponins show promise in lowering harmful cholesterol in your body by preventing your intestines from absorbing it, and this phytonutrient may even protect against colon cancer.[43] Eat legumes like chickpeas and soybeans to feel these health benefits.

Silymarin

Silymarin has anti-inflammatory and antioxidant abilities and may be helpful in reducing the growth of cancer cells.[44] Natural health practitioners use silymarin to help detoxify and strengthen the liver.

This phytonutrient is found primarily in artichokes and the seeds of the herb milk thistle.

Sulforaphane

The phytonutrient sulforaphane lowers blood levels of cancer-stimulating estrogens in as few as five days, according to the American Institute for Cancer Research. Sulforaphane halts the growth of cancer cells on contact by neutralizing cancer cells before they can damage your body's genetic material.[45] For people looking to lose weight, this powerful phytonutrient can increase weight loss by as much as 22 percent, according to research at Nashville's Vanderbilt University Medical Center.[46] It works by releasing trapped toxins that slow metabolism and increase fat storage within fat cells.

Sulforaphane is found in many foods, including bok choy, broccoli, brussels sprouts, cabbage, cauliflower, and other cruciferous vegetables, as well as dark leafy greens.

Tangeretin

Tangeretin has shown promise in lowering cholesterol, fighting cancer, and even protecting the brain against damage from Parkinson's disease. In one animal study, tangeretin reduced LDL cholesterol levels by up to 40 percent. And in laboratory tests, researchers found that tangeretin demonstrated antitumor activity against cancer tumors by encouraging leukemia cells to self-destruct without having any harmful effect on healthy cells. However, it seems to interfere with the cancer drug tamoxifen. In another animal study of Parkinson's disease, tangeretin increased the levels of the brain hormone dopamine and demonstrated brain protective activity.[47]

You can find tangeretin in the peels of lemons, oranges, and other citrus fruits. Now, I'm not suggesting that you eat the peel of these fruits all by themselves. But a small amount of the peel of organic citrus fruits grated into soups, stews, stir-fries, and other foods can offer excellent flavor and some health benefits too.

Tannins

Tannins show antibacterial activity, can help to ease diarrhea, and seem to have a protective effect on the body's genetic material. However, I do caution that you not consume tannins in high quantities, because they can interfere with your body's iron absorption.[48] Tannins are found in berries, the herb nettle, tea, and wine aged in oak barrels.

Terpene Limonoids

Numerous terpenes exist that offer health benefits, including limonoids. There are about 40 types of limonoids alone. Research shows that they have powerful anticancer activity and significantly improve the liver's ability to eliminate toxins we've inhaled or ingested, including cancer-causing agents.[49] They also demonstrate antiviral and cholesterol-lowering properties in studies.[50]

You can benefit from these phytonutrients by eating citrus fruits like grapefruit, lemons, limes, and oranges.

Zeaxanthin

Zeaxanthin shares some of the effects of lutein. Specifically, it is proven to prevent age-related macular degeneration, the leading cause of blindness in the elderly.[51] An interesting study found that high amounts of vitamins C and E, beta-carotene, cryptoxanthin, lutein, and zeaxanthin may protect against DNA damage caused from high amounts of radiation, particularly that associated with airplane travel.[52]

Eat yellow-orange foods like apricots, mangoes, and sweet potatoes to get more of this phytonutrient in your diet.

Phytonutrients for Your Unique Needs

In Part Two you'll learn about some of the best phytonutrients for specific health conditions. For those of you suffering from a particular health condition, I created the following table to help you quickly and simply identify some of the best phytonutrients for your needs. I encourage you to refer to the table often, so you can eat more of the foods that contain those beneficial substances. Sometimes improving your diet is as simple as eating more of the foods that are beneficial to you. By doing so, you'll automatically be eating fewer of the harmful foods.

Phytonutrients: What They Do and Where to Find Them		
Phytonutrient	Uses*	Primary Sources
Alpha-carotene	cancer, particularly lung cancer and breast cancer; eyesight; immunity	apricots, broccoli, carrots, collards, leafy greens, kale, mangoes, papayas, peaches, sweet potatoes, pumpkin, spinach, squash, tomatoes
Anthocyanins	aging, allergies, inflammatory conditions, obesity, excess weight	blackberries, blueberries, cherries, red grapes, raspberries, strawberries
Astaxanthin	arthritis; brain and nervous system protection; cancer, particularly liver cancer and colon cancer; cellular energy; diabetes-related conditions; heart disease; joint and muscle pain; liver damage; skin; sun damage to skin; wrinkling	carrots, red peppers, red-colored fruits and vegetables
Beta-carotene	aging, eyesight, immunity, skin	apricots, broccoli, carrots, collards, leafy greens, kale, mangoes, papayas, peaches, sweet potatoes, pumpkin, spinach, squash, tomatoes

Continued on page 32

Continued from page 31

Phytonutrients: What They Do and Where to Find Them		
Phytonutrient	**Uses***	**Primary Sources**
Beta-sitosterol	cancer, particularly breast cancer, colon cancer, and prostate cancer; high cholesterol	corn oil, flaxseed, peanuts, pumpkin seeds, rice bran, soybeans, wheat germ
Capsaicin	arthritis, gastric ulcer prevention, pain disorders, psoriasis	chili peppers
Catechins	blood sugar balancing, inflammatory conditions, obesity, skin health, excess weight	green and black tea
Chlorogenic acid	cancer, particularly liver cancer; diabetes; obesity; excess weight	apples, carrots, coffee, flaxseed, pineapple, potatoes, strawberries
Cryptoxan-thin	cancer, particularly cervical cancer	oranges, papayas, peaches, tangerines
Curcumin	aging, Alzheimer's disease, brain and nervous system conditions, inflammatory conditions, neurological pain disorders, pain disorders,	turmeric (spice)
Ellagic acid	cancer, DNA damage, liver detoxification	blackberries, blueberries, sweet and sour cherries, black and red currants, elderberries, grapes, raspberries, strawberries
Ferulic acid	high blood sugar, cancer, diabetes, DNA damage, skin damage from UV rays	brown rice, whole grains, whole wheat, wheat bran, blackberries, blueberries, sweet and sour cherries, coffee, black and red currants, elderberries, grapes, raspberries, strawberries

Hesperetin/ Hesperidin	allergies, cancer, high cholesterol, heart disease, inflammatory conditions, osteoporosis	citrus fruits like lemons and oranges, green vegetables
Indole-3-carbinol	cancer, particularly breast cancer, prostate cancer (still controversial), and skin cancer; heart disease	cruciferous vegetables: broccoli, brussels sprouts, cabbage, cauliflower, kale
Isoflavones	cancer, particularly breast cancer and prostate cancer; heart disease; menopause; metabolic syndrome; osteoporosis; stroke	chickpeas (garbanzo beans), miso, soybeans, tempeh, tofu
Lipoic acid	age-related diseases, fatigue, chronic fatigue syndrome, excess weight and obesity	dark leafy greens: collards, kale, spinach, Swiss chard
Lutein	Arteriosclerosis; eyesight, particularly age-related vision loss and macular degeneration; heart disease; stroke	apricots, avocados, broccoli, carrots, collards, eggs, leafy greens, kale, mangoes, papayas, peaches, sweet potatoes, pumpkin, spinach, squash, tomatoes
Lycopene	asthma; atherosclerosis; cancer, particularly pancreatic cancer, prostate cancer, and breast cancer; heart disease; hypertension; nervous system disorders; osteoporosis; radiation protection	guavas, pink grapefruit, papayas, rose hips, strawberries, tomatoes, watermelon
Naringin	brain injury, cancer, high cholesterol, eye disorders in diabetics, stroke	grapefruit
Perrillyl alcohol	cancer	cherries, mint

Continued on page 34

Continued from page 33

Phytonutrients: What They Do and Where to Find Them

Phytonutrient	Uses*	Primary Sources
Proanthocya-nidin	allergies; brain and nervous system protection against toxins; cancer, particularly breast cancer; heart disease	dark red- to purple-colored fruits like blueberries, cherries, cranberries grapes, raspberries, and strawberries, as well as almonds, apples, cocoa, peanuts
Quercetin	allergies; asthma; bronchitis; cancer, particularly prostate cancer, colon cancer, ovarian cancer, breast cancer, gastric cancer, lung cancer, and cervical cancer; lung disorders; rhinitis; sinusitis	apples, berries, cabbage, cauliflower, nuts, onions, tea
Resveratrol	Alzheimer's disease, brain disease, cancer, protection against chemotherapy, diabetes, protection against damage to genetic material, heart disease, inflammatory conditions, liver detoxification, stroke	blueberries, purple and red grapes, purple grape juice, mulberries, peanuts, red wine
Rutin	strengthens blood vessels, especially capillaries; circulatory disorders; diabetic retinopathy; eye disorders; heart disease; high cholesterol	citrus fruits, red apples, apricots, bilberry fruit, blackberries, broccoli, buckwheat, cherries, black currants, grapes, nuts, onions, peppers, plums, prunes, rose hips, tea
Saponins	cancer, particularly colon cancer; high cholesterol	chickpeas (garbanzo beans), soybeans
Silymarin	cancer, inflammatory conditions, liver conditions, liver detoxification	milk thistle seeds (herb)

Sulforaphane	cancer, particularly estrogen-dependent cancer and prostate cancer; liver detoxification; obesity; excess weight	bok choy, broccoli, broccoli sprouts, brussels sprouts, cabbage, cauliflower, other cruciferous vegetables, dark leafy greens, kale
Tangeretin	brain and nervous system disorders; cancer, particularly leukemia; high cholesterol; Parkinson's disease	the peels of citrus fruits like lemons, oranges, tangerines
Tannins	bacterial infections, bowel conditions, diarrhea, DNA	berries, nettle (herb), tea, wine aged in oak barrels
Terpene limonoids	cancer, high cholesterol, liver detoxification, viruses	citrus fruits like grapefruit, lemons, limes, oranges
Zeaxanthin	DNA damage, age-related macular degeneration	apricots, broccoli, carrots, collards, eggs, leafy greens, kale, mangoes, papayas, peaches, sweet potatoes, pumpkin, spinach, squash, tomatoes

This list is by no means exhaustive. As I said, exciting new research appears almost daily espousing benefits and new uses of phytonutrients.

Phytonutrients: A Rainbow of Healthful Choice

Part of maximizing great health is getting a broad spectrum of phyto-nutrients. So how do you know if you're getting enough? Simple. Eat a wide variety of fruits and vegetables and make a conscious effort to eat a whole range of colors every day. If you eat yellow-orange, red, green, and bluish-purple fruits and vegetables every day, you can feel confident that you're getting hundreds of phytonutrients that will not only impart their disease-prevention powers but also increase your well-being. For example, if in a day you drink a glass of water with fresh lemon juice, eat a plateful of salad greens topped with strawberries, enjoy roasted sweet potatoes, and drink a blueberry-banana almond-milk smoothie, you've covered all the colors of the phytonutrient rainbow.

Science and nutrition research have come a long way since Columbus's crew first discovered the power of vitamin C. But as we're seeing, there are still new areas to explore and new discoveries to be made. Thanks to the many pioneering researchers in the field of nutritional science over the last century, we know that many other nutrients can ensure our health, aid our fight against illness, and improve our quality of life.

While the research into phytonutrients is still in the exploration stage, we know that they share a common role as nature's healers. Not only do they help prevent countless diseases and reverse many illnesses, they strengthen immunity, boost energy, improve cellular functioning, slow the aging process, and help restore healthy and balanced weight as well.

This is just the beginning of the Phytozyme Cure. In the next chapter, you'll learn about enzymes and how they play a significant role not only in keeping you healthy, but also in healing many health conditions.

2
CHAPTER

Enzymes: The Building Blocks of Great Health

I learned that healing and cure are active processes in which I myself needed to participate.

—Rollo May

Most people are deficient in an important nutritional factor, making them overweight or obese, exhausted, and at risk for many health conditions. Some researchers even estimate that at least 80 percent of women have this deficiency, and I believe the percentage may be even higher among men. What nutritional factor are people missing? Enzymes.

If you're like most people, you probably aren't aware of the full power of enzymes. You may think that you only need them to digest food, but your body uses enzymes all the time. They are the sparks of every chemical reaction in your body, involved in everything from fighting a cold to killing cancer cells. And just like you need a spark to start a fire, you need enzymes to ensure that your body can perform its thousands of functions to keep you healthy and alive.

In this chapter, you'll discover why enzymes are essential to great health and how you can maximize your body's enzyme potential.

You'll also learn about some of the important roles enzymes play in your body.

Types of Enzymes

Each enzyme has a specialized function. For example, an enzyme that helps produce hormones cannot detoxify your body from chemicals you breathe in, and an enzyme that helps kill cancer cells cannot bind cholesterol and eliminate it from your body. However, some digestive enzymes can not only aid the digestion of specific types of foods like proteins, carbohydrates, or fats, they can also aid the healing of many health conditions in your body.

There are currently over five thousand known enzymes, and potentially thousands more we haven't discovered yet. They fall into three main categories: digestive, metabolic, and food enzymes. Although some do span multiple categories (which I'll talk about later), let's first take a look at the three main types of enzymes.

Digestive Enzymes

Digestive enzymes do exactly what you think: they assist with digestion. To be more specific, they assist with breaking down foods into nutrients so your body can absorb them properly. Digestive enzymes are also called pancreatic enzymes, because at least 22 kinds are manufactured and secreted by the pancreas—the organ under the lower left side of your rib cage that regulates your blood sugar levels. These essential enzymes include amylase, lipase, and protease, which digest carbohydrates, fats, and proteins respectively. But we'll discuss more about these enzymes in a moment.

The quantity of digestive enzymes determines how well your body will digest and absorb food nutrients. Digestion has many stages and involves many parts of your body, including your mouth, stomach, duodenum, pancreas, and the small and large intestines.

The duodenum connects the stomach and small intestines. Through ducts in the duodenum, enzymes from the pancreas and liver are secreted. If an insufficient amount of enzymes is secreted at any stage of digestion, the other organs have to work harder, and sometimes they simply cannot handle the load.

There are a few reasons why your body may not be producing enough digestive enzymes:

1. You're not chewing your food properly, so it doesn't break down as it mingles with saliva.
2. You're eating too much of a particular type of food, which puts a strain on your body's ability to manufacture the enzymes you need to digest this food.
3. You have impaired organ function, including reduced function of either the liver or pancreas.
4. You drink a lot with meals, which dilutes the enzymes and makes them less effective. It doesn't matter whether you're drinking water, juice, or alcohol, as they all dilute digestive enzymes.
5. You take a lot of antacids, which disrupts the pH balance of your stomach and causes food to reach your intestines too quickly, before your stomach's digestive juices have done their job.
6. You've had part of your digestive tract removed.
7. You've made unhealthy diet and lifestyle choices, such as smoking, drinking alcohol, overeating, overusing medications, or eating prepackaged foods containing additives like artificial flavors and colors.
8. You suffer from chronic stress, which can deplete enzymes or the nutrients they need to work.

Metabolic Enzymes

Your body makes metabolic enzymes to properly run all of its biochemical processes, from moving and talking to breathing and thinking. Each one of these enzymes has a unique function. A deficiency in any particular metabolic enzyme can lead to any number of serious diseases.

One type of metabolic enzyme that you may have heard about is a group called antioxidant enzymes. Some are similar to antioxidant nutrients like vitamins C and E, which we must ingest to get their benefits. But many are manufactured inside our bodies specifically to destroy free radicals, which are linked to many diseases and aging. A free radical is an atom or molecule with an unpaired electron. You may remember from science class that electrons surround the nucleus of an atom in pairs. A missing electron means the atom or molecule is positively charged and highly reactive. In our bodies, that spells trouble, as the free radical will seek out other molecules or atoms to steal an electron, creating more free radicals and wreaking havoc at the cellular level.

Free radicals form naturally during metabolism and your body is designed to combat them. But we're increasingly exposed to free radicals through toxins and chemicals in our air, food, and water. When our diet is low in antioxidants such as vitamin C, which destroy free radicals, our bodies must use substantial energy to manufacture antioxidant enzymes to keep up with the free radicals. This is an enormous task, as we are increasingly exposed to more free radicals and ingesting fewer antioxidant nutrients. If our bodies cannot keep pace with the free radicals, we sustain cellular damage, age faster, and are more prone to illness.

Perhaps doctors have overlooked enzymes because there has been confusion about the connection between this class of enzymes— metabolic enzymes—and digestive enzymes. While they assist with different bodily functions (the latter obviously aids digestion), they are both produced by the same organs—the pancreas and liver. We'll learn more about these important organs momentarily.

For now, it is important to understand that if our bodies don't have adequate amounts of digestive enzymes, the pancreas and liver shift their focus from creating essential metabolic enzymes needed for vital life functions to assisting with digestion. In other words, digesting food is such a significant function that if our body needs help breaking down food, we fall short in manufacturing critical enzymes for other metabolic processes. That's no surprise when you consider the vital importance of our bodies' ability to break down food into the building blocks of cells, hormones, tissues, glands, and organs.

So potentially thousands of life-supporting metabolic processes, including burning fat for energy, may suffer if there is a deficiency of enzymes in the body. And, you guessed it: this enzyme deficiency is linked, at least in part, to our current obesity and overweight epidemic.

Of the five thousand or so enzymes made in the body, approximately three thousand are manufactured by bacteria. We normally think of bacteria as harmful, but there are many beneficial bacteria in our bodies that we need to live. Actually, about half of your body's cells are bacterial, most of which are beneficial and inhabit the digestive system. The vast majority of these bacteria are striving to keep you healthy and play a vital role in the proper functioning of your body. We'll discuss more about the importance of beneficial bacteria and how to keep them functioning at their peak in Chapter 3.

Food Enzymes

Sometimes called plant enzymes, you can find food enzymes in raw plants such as fruits, vegetables, and herbs. Your body also manufactures some food enzymes to aid digestion and other bodily functions. So, by eating a diet rich in food enzymes, you will dramatically reduce the number of digestive enzymes your body needs to manufacture, freeing up energy and making more enzymes available to your body for healing. (To learn more about how to eat a diet rich in food enzymes, consult my book *The Life Force Diet*.) In addition to eating a diet rich in enzymes, supplementing with specific food enzymes at specific times and in specific quantities can not only assist with digestion but have enormous healing implications on many seemingly unrelated health conditions.

Yet, due to food processing and heating techniques used in preparing food, enzymes are almost completely depleted from our food supply. According to research presented by prominent enzyme researcher Dr. Ellen Cutler, 70 percent of American women get almost no enzymes in their diet.[1] And I would estimate that at least the same number may apply to men. Actually, many men are more likely to avoid fruits and vegetables and forgo responsible eating for a diet rich in enzyme-deficient cooked meat and processed fare. It makes sense that they would also be at risk of enzyme depletion.

First for Women magazine conducted an interview with Joseph Brasco, a gastroenterologist at the Center for Colon and Digestive Disease in Huntsville, Alabama. In the interview he discussed the way in which a lack of enzymes derived from food forces the liver and pancreas to use energy creating digestive enzymes to break down a meal. He added: "Because the pancreas and liver need energy to produce enzymes, the resulting drain renders these organs temporarily unable to perform their functions of detoxification, blood sugar control, and fat burning."[2] And that's just the start. The result of the impairment of just these three functions can lead us to feel exhausted, suffer from mood swings, become overweight, or, over the longer term, become more vulnerable to chronic illness like heart disease, diabetes, and cancer. And with five hundred other functions for just the liver to perform, this overworked organ needs all the energy it can muster.

As I said earlier, your pancreas manufactures and secretes approximately 22 digestive enzymes into the upper part of the small intestine where they continue to digest food after plant enzymes started working on it earlier in the digestive process. Amylase helps digest starchy foods, also called carbohydrates. Lipase digests fatty foods. Proteases, which are also sometimes called proteolytic enzymes, are responsible for digesting proteins in foods. You can also find these three primary types of enzymes in certain foods under the right conditions, as you'll find out in a moment.

According to research by one of the earliest enzymologists, Dr. Edward Howell, enzyme shortages are commonly seen in people suffering from chronic diseases, including allergies, premature aging, some forms of cancer, heart disease, skin conditions, and obesity.[3]

More recently, many natural health experts have found that specific types of enzymes have been successfully used to treat and, in some cases, even reverse many illnesses.

Clinical data collected by Hiromi Shinya, MD, clinical professor of surgery at Albert Einstein College of Medicine, shows a correlation between the levels of enzymes in people's diets and the amount of bodily enzymes they have.[4] This is incredible research because it means that our diet is far more important than we may have ever realized. It suggests that the quantity of enzymes we ingest through food and supplementation can play a role in determining the amount of internal bodily enzymes we have available for essential functions. To help you understand this important research, let's further explore the role of particular enzymes in your food.

As I mentioned earlier, amylase digests starches, lipase digests fats, and proteases digest proteins. All of these enzymes are found in foods containing these nutritional building blocks. For example, fatty foods naturally contain enough lipase to help digest them. Unfortunately, most enzymes, lipase included, are destroyed at temperatures of 118 degrees Fahrenheit, which is a substantially lower temperature than most cooking, canning, packaging, or other types of food processing entails. So, the enzymes that help to digest this food are eliminated and your body must compensate by manufacturing the enzymes needed for this task. And, not all the enzymes found in food can be manufactured by your body, and vice versa. For example, fibrous foods like fruits, vegetables, nuts, and seeds contain the enzyme cellulase that digests the soluble fiber that these foods contain. If those enzymes are destroyed or the cellular walls surrounding them insufficiently broken down through chewing, then your body may struggle to digest these foods because it cannot manufacture cellulase.

The Amazing Healing Power of Enzymes

Our bodies use enzymes in vast quantities to quell inflammation, promote wound healing, and regenerate tissues, all of which are essential processes involved in healing most chronic illnesses.

Our immune system's ability to fight off foreign invaders appears to be linked to the enzyme protease that helps digest proteins in foods. However, it is involved in much more than digestion. The enzyme that digests protein in your foods, if present in sufficient quantities when there is no food to work on, will literally digest bodily invaders. This is because most immune system invaders are proteins or have protein outer structures. Even cancer cells are coated with a protein called fibrin that can be broken down by supplementary protease. Research shows that blood clots linked to stroke and heart attacks are made up of this protein.[5]

In his book *Everything You Need to Know About Enzymes,* Tom Bohager cites research that shows the greater burden we place on the digestive system, the less effective and active our immune system becomes. He aptly states:

The protease production so essential to immune support decreases since the energy required to manufacture these enzymes has been dedicated to producing digestive enzymes. We pay the price initially by being tired, but over time by suffering from poor health. If the pattern persists over years, our body may no longer be able to keep up on a regular basis; a shortage of certain metabolic enzymes [metabolic energy] will then occur, and eventually take its toll. However, we do not call it an enzyme deficiency—we have given it other names like diabetes, cancer, heart disease, and lupus.[6]

Dr. Anthony Cichoke cites exciting information about the effects of enzymes on rheumatoid arthritis in his book *Enzymes & Enzyme Therapy.* He indicates that rheumatoid arthritis improves or is at least delayed when high doses of enzymes are used over an extended period of time.[7]

Other research shows the tremendous promise enzymes offer to sufferers of HIV (human immunodeficiency virus). According to AVERT, an international HIV charity, an estimated 33.2 million people are currently suffering from HIV, including the 1.3 million sufferers of this tragic disease in North America.[8] According to research in Germany and Puerto Rico, the use of enzymes to treat these illnesses is having positive results.[9]

In one study exploring the presence of lipase in overweight and obese individuals, researchers indicate that they believe overweight and obesity may be linked to a lipase (fat-digesting) enzyme deficiency. The study found that 100 percent of clinically obese individuals (those whose weight is more than 30 percent greater than the ideal weight) were deficient in lipase.[10]

While we cannot supplement directly with metabolic enzymes, we can increase the enzymes in our food and supplement with particular food and digestive enzymes that have a therapeutic effect. You can take enzyme supplements with meals to improve digestion (and therefore nutrient absorption) and on an empty stomach to work on other substances in your body, including bacteria, fungi, yeasts, parasites, inflammation, cancer cells, dead or damaged cells, or other contributors to disease.

Enzymes and Inflammation

Enzymes are particularly valuable in alleviating inflammation, which is now being linked to most chronic diseases and premature aging. Sometimes inflammation can be beneficial to clean up wounds, attack viruses, and for other good purposes in the body. But when your immune system becomes overactive, it can attack even seemingly harmless substances in your blood. Or inflammation can become chronic, which can prevent healing of injured or damaged areas. In these situations, enzymes can support and accelerate your body's natural inflammatory processes, while stopping it from getting out of control.

Because there are many chronic inflammatory conditions (including arthritis, lupus, prostate enlargement, sinus infections, diabetes, sports or traumatic injuries, lupus and other autoimmune disorders, to name a few) enzymes have almost endless applications. Due to their ability to accelerate the body's natural inflammatory processes without allowing it to go uncontrolled, enzymes can help the body regulate inflammation. Enzymes work on inflammation on four levels, including:[11]

1. Breaking down proteins in the blood (called circulating immune complexes) that cause inflammation, and encouraging their removal in the blood and lymphatic systems. The lymphatic system is a complex network of fluid-filled nodes, glands, and tubes that bathe our cells and carry the body's "sewage" away from the tissues and neutralize it. It comprises lymph glands, nodes, spleen, thymus, and tonsils, as well as vessels and ducts. These elements of the lymph system work together to carry cellular waste to the bloodstream. It handles toxins that enter your body from external sources such as foods or air pollution but also handles internally produced toxins (endotoxins) that are the result of normal metabolic processes—one example is inflammation. The lymph system helps carry the waste products of inflammation to your blood to be eliminated.

2. Removing fibrin, the clotting material that prolongs inflammation—sometimes excessively.

3. Clearing up excess water (edema) in the injured or inflamed areas where inflammation exists.

4. Counteracting chronic, long-standing, or recurrent inflammation that can be linked to chronic degenerative conditions like arthritis.

Substantial amounts of research show that, in many circumstances, enzymes are more effective than nonsteroidal anti-inflammatory drugs (NSAIDs). They may take longer for people to notice symptom improvement, but the improvement will usually be more effective, more complete, and without the side effects and long-term organ damage that often accompanies drugs. Enzymes also appear to accelerate the healing process.[12]

There is even research that shows enzyme supplements may reduce physical stress in athletes who follow challenging training regimens. Dr. Wolfgang Bringmann and Dr. Rudolf Kunze, of Berlin, conducted a study of athletes at an official mini-marathon. For two days prior to the event Dr. Bringmann gave the athletes 10 enzyme tablets three times per day. On the morning of the event, the athletes took 10 additional enzyme supplements. The athletes maintained their strict training schedules throughout this test. Dr. Kunze took blood samples of the athletes and observed that the levels of lymphocytes, a substance created by the body as part of an immune system response typically indicating physical stress, were remarkably reduced, which indicated that the athletes' bodies were less stressed by their physical activity.

Enzymes and Immune System Disorders

In many immune system disorders, the immune system malfunctions and goes into a hyperactive state. It overreacts to many common substances, causing environmental or food sensitivities or allergies, or the body may even begin to attack its own tissues and organs. The latter can be serious, debilitating, and even potentially life-threatening. So any substance that improves the body's ability to regulate the immune response has tremendous therapeutic potential. Research shows that enzymes have a regulatory effect on the immune system.[13]

Consider rheumatoid arthritis, a painful and debilitating condition in which the immune system attacks the body's joints. In a study published in the German journal *Zeitschrift für Rheumatologie,* 62 percent of patients taking a particular enzyme formulation called Wobenzym N showed improvement. Another study found that the same enzyme formula prevented further arthritic flare-ups and lowered inflammatory compounds called circulating immune complexes.

But rheumatoid arthritis isn't the only type of arthritis in which enzymes are showing great promise. In one study of patients suffering from osteoarthritis, people were given either Wobenzym N or the nonsteroidal anti-inflammatory drug diclofenac, or a placebo. After evaluating all principal symptom criteria, the enzyme formulation demonstrated equivalent therapeutic results as diclofenac.[14] Wobenzym N has also demonstrated positive effects in the treatment of children suffering from chronic hepatitis.[15]

Treating Inflammation with Enzymes[16]

Amylase is the enzyme that helps us to digest carbohydrates. When you take it on an empty stomach it has antihistamine effects and alleviates inflammation linked to skin conditions, particularly when combined with lipase. Amylase is also well suited for athletes because it increases joint mobility and relieves muscle pain and inflammation.[17]

Bromelain is helpful in treating swelling and inflammation that is linked to injuries, surgery, swellings, and broken blood vessels; menstrual hemorrhaging; and blood clots.[18]

Catalase helps relieve inflammation linked to injuries, particularly when fluid-retention and edema are involved. This enzyme also functions as an antioxidant, which scavenges free radicals and prevents them from causing additional health concerns.

Chymotrypsin is effective in treating inflammation, abscesses, wounds, and blood clots before and after tooth extractions and other dental work, as well as after surgeries.

Lipase is particularly good for alleviating lymphatic swelling, and muscle spasms linked to a calcium deficiency.

Papain is helpful against insect stings and can help treat inflammation linked to gluten intolerance, swelling, and wounds.

Protease supplementation is excellent for inflammation that tends to benefit from ice packs. It also alleviates soft tissue trauma linked to accidents or surgery. Like lipase, protease is also good for muscle spasms if they are linked to a calcium deficiency.

Trypsin is helpful for treating wounds, abscesses, blood clots, injuries, and inflammations.

Enzymes and Cancer

Enzymes have been used for many years in Europe to treat cancer and numerous other diseases. In an effort to establish policy on enzymes for cancer treatment, the European Union commissioned extensive studies. Researchers examined the effectiveness of enzymes as cancer treatment or as a complementary treatment for various types of cancer and concluded that "these studies demonstrated that enzyme therapy significantly decreased tumor-induced and therapy-induced side effects and complaints such as nausea, gastrointestinal complaints, fatigue, weight loss, and restlessness and obviously stabilized the quality of life." For some types of cancer "enzyme therapy was shown to increase the response rates, the duration of (cancer) remissions, and the overall survival times."[19]

Enzyme therapy has demonstrated its effectiveness in breast and bone cancer treatment.[20,21] It has also been effective following breast cancer surgery to alleviate arm swelling.[22] Enzymes have been helpful in preventing the fibrous changes in the lungs, skin, fatty tissue, soft tissue, liver, and kidneys, which are linked to radiation treatment for lung, cervical, breast, and lymphatic cancers.[23]

In a study of mice, the enzyme bromelain (found in pineapples) was able to prevent skin cancer. This may be because bromelain literally digests the outer protein membrane of the cancer cells, so the immune system can recognize cancer cells and kill them more effectively.[24] In another animal study, animals with cancer that was treated with three types of enzymes—chymotrypsin, trypsin, and papain—lived substantially longer than animals which did not receive enzyme therapy.[25] Similar results were found in research studying pancreatic and breast cancers in humans.[26]

Research at the Memorial Sloan-Kettering Cancer Center in New York City found the enzyme bromelain showed positive effects on the immune system. The researchers indicate that the improvements in immune system markers may help explain some of the clinical effects they've observed following bromelain treatment in patients suffering from chronic inflammatory disease, HIV, and cancer.[27]

Life Extension and Enzyme Potential

Enzymes are not only showing tremendous promise in the treatment of illness, they may even help us live longer. Let me explain a bit more about the nature of enzymes to help you understand their link to longevity.

Enzymes are the ultimate philanthropists. They give all of their energy to perform their specific biological activity until they are completely exhausted. At that point they become like any other protein in the body and are absorbed.

The traditional school of thought on enzymes was that the body had unlimited quantities to ensure the proper functioning of every bodily process, under almost any circumstance, for as long as we lived. However, newer research indicates that we have a limited number of enzymes that must last throughout our lifetime.

Dr. Edward Howell coined the term "enzyme potential" during his many years of research on enzymes that culminated in his book *Enzyme Nutrition*. He says that our enzyme potential is the number of enzymes we have the ability to produce in our bodies during our lifetime. He proposed the concept that our lifespan was linked to our enzyme potential, and that once we used up our potential to create enzymes, our lives would end.

There is still debate among scientists and nutritionists as to whether this theory is accurate, but it is proving to be valid. Roy Walfor, MD, reduced the daily food intake of mice in his laboratory at UCLA (thereby reducing the enzymes required for digesting the food) and observed that the mice lived 25 percent longer than controls. There are no lifelong human studies that confirm a link between reduced caloric intake and increased lifespan. But short-term trials indicate that eating less is linked to reduced body weight and healthier levels of blood pressure, cholesterol, and blood glucose—all of which are risk factors for two major killers: heart disease and diabetes.[28] There is still debate in the scientific community over the link between reduced food volume and increased longevity, but I believe it may be due to the reduced demands on the body to manufacture enzymes for digestion.

Now, I'm not going to suggest that you substantially reduce the volume of food you ingest every day. But by increasing the amount of enzyme-rich food you eat, you will reduce the amount of enzymes your body must manufacture to digest food, thereby achieving "metabolic efficiency"—the concept Dr. Walfor proposed based on the results of his study. And not only does increasing enzymes in our foods have the potential to increase our lifespan, it has the power to improve our quality of life, as you will learn momentarily.

The Conditions Needed for Enzymes to Work

Simply eating enzyme-rich food is not enough to ensure you are getting enzymes in your diet. Enzymes are something of nutritional prima donnas: they require very specific conditions to do their work, or they simply won't work at all. Some enzymes are stimulated by the presence of hormones or biochemical regulators. They can also be inhibited by the by-products of metabolism. These by-products build up, which stops enzyme production until the buildup is reduced or depleted.

Not having the right substances or coenzymes—nutrients that function as assistants to enzymes—that enzymes need to work can also inhibit their function. External factors such as viruses, drugs, vitamins, and foreign chemicals can stimulate or inhibit activity. In additional, enzymes are stimulated by many factors, including specific temperature range, pH levels, and moisture. Other factors, such as the temperatures at which you cook your food, medications you take, and having certain heavy metals in your body, can also interfere with the way enzymes work. Even how much you chew—or don't chew—your food can affect an enzyme's function. I'll tell you more about these factors a bit later on in this chapter.

A pHine Balancing Act

If you have ever used the natural cleaning products baking soda and vinegar, you already have some insight into pH. The term "pH" stands for "potential of hydrogen," which is the measure of acidity or alkalinity on a scale of zero to 14. Zero is the most acidic reading while 14 is the most alkaline reading. At the mid-point (7) you'll find neutral—a complete balance between acid and alkaline. Vinegar is highly acidic, while baking soda is alkaline. If you've poured baking soda down a drain and added vinegar, you'll have watched the two fizzle. They are chemically reacting to balance each other's acidity and alkaline levels to obtain neutrality.

Most of your body, your blood included, needs to be slightly alkaline. In the blood, the ideal is 7.365. When we eat highly acid-forming foods like meat, poultry, dairy products, sugar, and sweets, among others, our bodies have to deal with excess acid. This not only strains the detoxification mechanisms, it is a burden to the body's alkaline mineral reserves and could potentially weaken bones and muscles.

Enzymes in our bodies require a fairly balanced pH, erring on the side of alkalinity. If our bodies become too acidic, primarily through an acid-forming diet, chronic stress, a lack of exercise, and toxic exposures, then our bodies manufacture fewer enzymes. And the enzymes our bodies do manufacture may not work properly or at all. The more acidic our bodies are, the less effective our enzyme activity. Not only does this affect digestion, it affects almost every bodily function.

Drugs and Toxins

Medications and toxins that we're exposed to in our food, air, and water supply can interfere with enzymes by throwing off our bodies' delicate pH balance, depleting critical nutrients needed as coenzymes or enzyme cofactors, or by directly inhibiting the action of enzymes. I'm not suggesting that you discontinue your medications. Just be aware that you may have a greater need to eat a higher proportion of enzyme-rich foods like those I tell you about throughout this book. Always consult with your physician if you want to stop taking or lessen your dose of prescription medications.

The Temperature's Rising

Plant enzymes need the temperature to fall between 92 and 104 degrees Fahrenheit to work; otherwise they will be rendered ineffective or be destroyed. In other words, body temperature provides the ideal amount of heat for enzymes to begin their work. When it comes to enzymes in food, they cannot survive temperatures higher than 118 degrees Fahrenheit. Beyond that, they are destroyed.

The Need for Moisture

Enzymes found in plant foods must have moisture to function properly. Water molecules are required for enzymes to break apart molecular bonds in the food. So, in our bodies, saliva serves this purpose perfectly. Ensuring that you drink enough water throughout the day helps to provide the moisture needed for the many enzyme-mediated biochemical reactions to take place in your body.

Toxins and Heavy Metals

Many toxins and heavy metals, once inside our bodies, can interfere with the capacity of enzymes to work. For example, the heavy metals lead and mercury bind to various groups of proteins, and as I mentioned earlier, enzymes are a special type of protein. Once these metals bind to an enzyme, they do one of three things to it: (1) denature the enzyme; (2) inhibit the enzyme's ability to function at all; or (3) denature and inhibit the enzyme. The result can be disastrous—degenerative diseases, nerve damage, or potentially even death.[29]

Unfortunately, we're more exposed to toxins and heavy metals than ever before, thanks largely to the Industrial Revolution and our extensive use of these harmful substances in manufacturing and industry. You frequently find lead and mercury in food, particularly junk food and packaged food, making it increasingly important to eliminate these health-destroyers from your diet (and I'll explain how in the next chapter). Lead is found in water supplies fed by lead pipes in older homes, refined chocolate, canned food, as well as cigarette smoke, glossy and colored newsprint, and leaded candle wicks. Mercury typically finds its way into our bodies through immunizations as a preservative or through farmed fish or fish known to contain high levels of mercury, such as king mackerel, shark, swordfish, tilefish, tuna, and farmed salmon. Metal amalgam dental fillings contain high levels of mercury that vaporize in the presence of hot or acidic foods. So if you have these types of fillings, you could inhale mercury into your bloodstream.

Chew, Chew, Chew

Some enzymes—for example, cellulases—won't work in your body unless they've been released through chewing your food well. The action of chewing helps to liberate the enzymes from the surrounding food cells so they can better digest the food itself.

Discover Your Phytozyme Cure Type

Over many years of research and observation in clinical practice, I noticed similarities between some people's symptoms and their dietary patterns. Further research suggested that other health professionals shared these observations. It appeared that either as a result of inherent enzyme weaknesses or overconsumption of particular types of foods, people experienced certain health conditions or symptoms of illness. From my research, I concluded that people with digestive difficulties fall into four main types: those who have difficulty digesting carbohydrates, those who have trouble digesting fats, those who have problems digesting proteins, and those who have digestive issues with all of these foods.[30]

It seems that consuming more and more cooked, enzyme-deprived foods takes its toll on our bodies' own digestive enzymes, leaving fewer enzyme stores available for other functions outside of digestion. Combined with our tendency to gravitate toward the same types of foods, we deplete some enzymes more than others. For example, people who eat a lot of sweets, pastas, or breads tend to deplete the enzymes needed to digest these foods. People who follow high-protein diets tend to deplete the enzymes needed to digest those foods.

In Chapter 4, you'll learn about the different Phytozyme Cure Types: Carbohydrate, Fat, Protein, and Combination. You'll also discover the symptoms linked with each biochemical weakness, so you can see if you may be experiencing an enzyme deficiency. And, of course, I'll show you how to address your particular weakness through diet and supplementation. But first, let's explore the basic ways to replenish your enzyme supplies.

Healing with Enzymes

There are various ways to replenish your enzyme stores and heal your body using enzymes:

1. Eat more enzyme-rich food to reduce the energy burden on your body's digestive system.
2. Supplement with enzymes at mealtimes to improve digestion (and therefore the absorption of important nutrients found in food).
3. Supplement with specific enzymes away from food on an empty stomach so that the enzymes work on microbes, inflammation, cancer cells, or other unwanted substances.

Eating Enzyme-Rich Food

Eating food that contains plentiful amounts of enzymes is a good way to assist your body with its healing efforts. Enzyme-rich foods include those that have not been cooked, canned, processed, or otherwise altered. Foods can be heated up to 118 degrees Fahrenheit before the enzymes are destroyed; however, most cooking techniques go well above that temperature. Most packaged and processed foods are heated to extremely high temperatures, which means their enzymes are destroyed long before you put them in your shopping cart. Canned and jarred foods have been heated to high temperatures to prevent their spoilage.

Fruits, vegetables, nuts, seeds, and sprouts, in their unadulterated state, contain enzymes to assist with their digestion. Once chewed, these foods pass through a tube called the esophagus until it reaches the stomach. The first part is like a holding tank where the enzymes in the food that were released by chewing the food can continue working. Food spends approximately 30 to 45 minutes in the upper part of the stomach, where it continues to digest prior to moving along to the lower part of the stomach, where pepsin and hydrochloric acid are secreted to break down any protein in the food. Most people are surprised to learn that most fruits and vegetables contain protein, but it is true.

Stomaching Enzymes

Whenever I write about enzymes or explain them to people, someone always argues that enzymes can't possibly be beneficial, because they're destroyed or simply digested in the stomach. Even if this statement were true (it's not), people would still benefit from eating foods rich in enzymes and supplementing with additional enzymes.

While this argument against enzymes is commonplace, it is inaccurate for a couple of reasons. First, as you learned above, food sits in the upper part of the stomach for up to 45 minutes. During this time, any enzymes in the food work to digest the food even before it moves to the lower part of the stomach.

Second, enzymes require a certain pH range to function. The specific range depends on the enzyme in question. The acid in the stomach measures between two and three on the pH scale. In other words, strongly acidic. Enzymes that are derived from animal sources (chymotrypsin, pancreatin, and trypsin) are extracted from the pancreas, small intestines, and stomachs of animals, namely cows and pigs. These enzymes require an alkaline environment to function. So, manufacturers of enzyme supplements give these enzymes an "enteric coating" that enables them to survive intact in the stomach and then break down in the small intestine where the enzymes begin to work. An enteric coating is like a shield against acidity, helping to ensure the enzymes remain intact while in the lower chamber of the stomach.

As for vegetarian sources of enzymes, either found in the food you eat or in vegetarian-based enzyme supplements, most work in a broader pH range, including a highly acidic environment. Research proves that most plant-based enzymes survive stomach acid intact. In one study, researchers collected samples of a meal during various stages of the digestive process. They tested a meal without digestive enzymes under ideal digestive conditions, the same meal with digestive enzymes under ideal digestive conditions, the same meal without digestive enzymes and with a 70 percent reduction in gastric and intestinal secretions, and the same meal with digestive enzymes and with the same digestive impairment. Samples were assessed for glucose and nitrogen content to demonstrate both carbohydrate and protein digestion. In the study, the addition of enzymes improved the availability of both proteins and carbohydrates, regardless of whether digestion was ideal or impaired. Glucose from carbohydrates increased four times in the ideal digestive environment and seven times in the impaired digestive process with the addition of enzymes, over the meal without enzymes added. And proteins were twice the amount in the impaired digestive system with enzymes, over the one without the enzymes.[31] These numbers indicate that plant-based enzymes survive intact in stomach acidity.

Even enzymes that require an alkaline environment to work typically remain inactive while in the stomach acid until they reach an alkaline environment in the intestines, where they become activated.

Supplementing with Enzymes

One of the easiest ways to benefit from enzymes is to take a full-spectrum enzyme supplement at mealtimes to help digest food and absorb important nutrients. While there are many different enzyme supplements on the market, most of them contain the following enzymes: amylase to digest starches, cellulose to digest fiber, lipase to digest fats, and protease to digest proteins. Sometimes, manufacturers also add enzymes to digest sugars like sucrose (from cane sugar), lactose (from milk), and maltose (from grains).

Start by taking 1 capsule or tablet with every meal and snack to aid digestion. Even if you think your digestion is fine, you'll benefit from taking digestive enzyme supplements by

1. improving nutrient absorption,
2. allowing your body to use its own digestive enzymes for other essential functions that we discussed above, and
3. increasing energy, since your body won't have to manufacture as many enzymes for digestion.

If you have any digestive discomfort, bloating, heaviness, or other difficulty, increase the amount of digestive enzymes you take to 2 or 3 with each meal.

For more information on the most common digestive enzymes and how they help digestion, see the "Common Enzymes at a Glance" box, below. As you'll learn in the next chapter, you can supplement with these enzymes to assist digestion. Most manufacturers formulate a single supplement to contain all or most of the enzymes mentioned.

Common Enzymes at a Glance

Amylase: Breaks down polysaccharides into disaccharides, which simply means that they turn complex carbohydrates into simple sugars. "Poly" means many, "saccharide" means sugar, and "di" means two.

Cellulase: Breaks apart the bonds found in plant fiber, called cellulose, to release another form of glucose to fuel the body.

Disaccharidase: Breaks down sugars that are made up of two sugar molecules, for example, sucrose (from cane sugar), lactose (from milk), and maltose (from grains), into basic sugar molecules.

Lipase: Breaks fats (called triglycerides) into individual fatty acids and a substance called glycerol. When the body burns fat for energy, it releases both fatty acids and glycerol into the blood stream. Enzymes in the liver use glucose to provide energy for cellular metabolism. This is one of the essential fuels for smooth-running cells.

Protease: Breaks down the lengthy protein molecules into smaller amino acid chains and then eventually into individual amino acids.

In addition to taking enzymes with meals, taking them on an empty stomach has many healing benefits. Enzymes tend to be single-minded. For example, a protease enzyme will work on protein foods if they are found in the presence of the enzyme. But, when there is no food to digest, the enzyme diverts its attention to other functions. In the case of protease, they may divert their attention to microbes affecting your immune system, inflammation, or cancer cells, since their cells all have protein-based outer coatings.

I've mentioned some of the exciting research into the use of enzymes to aid healing of arthritis, cancer, HIV, and sports injuries, among other illnesses, as well as to aid longevity. These are some of the healing functions enzymes can have when they are taken away from meals. They go to work on the areas of the body that need their assistance, while leaving healthy tissue intact.

Animal- and Vegetarian-Source Enzyme Supplements

So which enzymes should you choose? While there are many types of enzymes, there are really only two main types of enzyme supplements: animal source or vegetarian source. Both have benefits. First, let's explore animal-source enzymes.

Animal-source enzymes include the enzymes pancreatin, trypsin, and chymotrypsin. There is extensive research into the role these enzymes play in various health conditions, including cancer. Chymotrypsin is excellent at reducing swelling and inflammation, aids arthritis and injuries, and helps eliminate intestinal worms and cancer. Pancreatin assists digestion and is helpful in the treatment of cystic fibrosis. Trypsin aids the pancreas in its functions, reduces bowel obstructions, and helps the body in the removal of dead tissue. It also reduces inflammation and allergic reactions, and helps to treat many illnesses, including arthritis, eczema, asthma, and urinary tract infections.

These types of enzymes tend to work in a smaller pH range than vegetarian-based enzymes. As a result, many manufacturers give them a special coating to help ensure they survive the acidity of the stomach intact. This coating is called enteric-coating.

Most types of enzymes used therapeutically are vegetarian-based. An example I gave earlier is the enzyme bromelain, which is extracted from pineapples. The enzyme papain is extracted from papayas. There are many other vegetarian enzymes that are useful for healing.

On page 62 you'll find a chart I've compiled to help you understand some of the most potent healing enzymes and their specific uses.

Safety and Side Effects of Enzyme Supplementation

Taking enzyme supplements is safe, and very few people experience side effects. You may notice a short-term change in the color and odor of your stools. You may also find that you experience an increased frequency of bowel movements and a tendency toward being more regular. Occasionally, some people will experience flatulence, fullness, nausea, or diarrhea. However, most people actually notice improvements in these areas if there were pre-existing issues. Like any food or drug, the rare person may have an allergic reaction, usually quite minor and only while using extremely high doses of enzymes. Most allergies are actually helped by enzyme supplementation. But, of course, everyone is different.

There are no reported long-term side effects or health concerns arising from the use of enzyme supplementation. In fact, most people actually experience improvements in their condition. Supplementing with enzymes, however, is not for everyone. If any of the following conditions apply to you, avoid taking enzyme supplements:

- You have a hereditary blood clotting disorder like hemophilia.
- You are undergoing dialysis.
- You are about to undergo surgery or have recently had surgery.
- You are using anticoagulant drugs or therapy.
- You are allergic to pork, in which case you should avoid enzymes from porcine sources.
- You are pregnant or lactating. There simply isn't sufficient research to indicate whether there may be any issues for pregnant or lactating women or their babies.

Common Enzymes and Their Functions[32,33]

Enzyme	Type	Function and Properties	Unit of Measure
Alpha-galactosidase (commonly sold under the brand name Beano)	Carbohydrate-digesting	Breaks down carbohydrates like raffinose, stachyose, and verbascose Reduces gas linked to eating a high-fiber diet including beans, vegetables, and grains	Galactosidase units (GALUs)
Amylase	Carbohydrate-digesting	Breaks down carbohydrates, including starch and glycogen Reduces food cravings Increases blood sugar Regulates histamine when taken on an empty stomach	Dextrinizing units (DUs) and Sanstedt Kneen Blish units (SKBUs)
Beta-glucanase	Carbohydrate-digesting	Breaks down carbohydrates, particularly glucan, which is found in barley, oats, and wheat	Beta-glucanase units (BGUs)
Bromelain	Protein-digesting	Breaks down protein Acts as an anti-inflammatory Can be used in place of pepsin or trypsin to treat digestive difficulties Treats cellulite, diabetic ulcers, boils, lung swelling Speeds recovery from injuries caused by trauma, sports, childbirth, and surgery, including sprains, strains, contusions Reduces swelling Treats sinusitis, bronchitis, pneumonia, and other respiratory disorders	Gelatin digesting units (GDUs) and Food Chemical Codex Papain units (FCCPUs)

Continued on page 64

Enzyme	Type	Benefits	Measured in
		Helps with arthritis and bone and joint disorders, cardiovascular conditions Boosts the immune system Aids body in identifying and destroying viruses and bacteria Helps fight cancer Helps allergies, infections, painful periods, thyroid conditions, intestinal bacterial conditions	
Catalase	Protein-digesting	Potent antioxidant that breaks down hydrogen peroxide into water and oxygen in the body May lower high cholesterol	Baker units
Cellulase	Carbohydrate-digesting	Breaks down cellulose in plant foods and chitin—a fiber found in the wall of yeasts (including *Candida albicans*) Breaks down cell walls to free nutrients in fruits and vegetables	Cellulase units (CUs)
Chymotrypsin	Protein-digesting	Breaks down protein Anti-inflammatory Reduces swelling Helps arthritis Benefits healing of soft tissue injuries, sprains, contusions, infection, edema Helps with abscesses and liquefying mucous to aid secretion Can be helpful for intestinal worms Used for cancer	Milligrams (mg) or United States Pharmacopeia (USP)

Continued from page 63

Common Enzymes and Their Functions[32,33]

Enzyme	Type	Function and Properties	Unit of Measure
Glucoamylase	Carbohydrate-digesting	Breaks down carbohydrates, particularly polysaccharides, which are long-chained carbohydrates	Amygalactosidase units (AGUs)
Hemicellulase	Carbohydrate-digesting	Breaks down carbohydrates, particularly polysaccharides	Hemicellulase units (HCUs)
Invertase (sucrase)	Carbohydrate-digesting	Breaks down carbohydrates, particularly sucrose and maltose, found in cane sugar and grains respectively	Invertase active units (IAUs)
Lactase	Carbohydrate-digesting	Breaks down milk sugar (lactose) Used to treat lactose intolerance	Lactase units (LacUs)
Lipase	Fat-digesting	Breaks down fats and improves fat utilization Helps lower cholesterol Supports weight loss Supports hormone production Supports gallbladder function	Food Chemical Codex Fédération Internationale Pharmaceutique (FCCFIP) and Lipase units (LUs)
Maltase (diastase and malt diastase)	Carbohydrate-digesting	Breaks down carbohydrates, particularly grain sugars and malt	Degrees of diastatic power (DP)
Mucolase	Protein-digesting	Breaks down mucus Helpful for congestion and sinus infections	Milligrams (mg) or Mucolase units (MSUs)

Continued on page 66

Nattokinase	Protein-digesting	Breaks down fibrin, a protein that forms in the blood to aid clotting after injuries or traumas; and toxins; helpful for infections in the blood Helps treat cardiovascular conditions, circulation problems, high blood pressure	Fibrinolytic units (FUs)
Pancreatin	Protein-, carbohydrate-, and fat-digesting due to rich enzyme content (mainly trypsin, chymotrypsin, amylase, and lipase)	Breaks down protein, fats, and carbohydrates Aids absorption of nutrients in food Used to treat cystic fibrosis	Milligrams (mg) or United States Pharmacopeia (USP)
Papain	Protein-digesting	Breaks down protein Anti-inflammatory Works similarly to chymotrypsin Diuretic Useful for allergies, hay fever, and catarrh Treats infections and infected wounds, sores, ulcers, tumors Aids chronic diarrhea and celiac disease Treats intestinal parasites Treats soft tissue injuries, including strains, sprains, contusions, pulled muscles, sports injuries	Food Chemical Codex Papain units (FCCPUs)

Continued from page 65

Common Enzymes and Their Functions[32,33]

Enzyme	Type	Function and Properties	Unit of Measure
		Used in creams to exfoliate skin	
		Useful to treat surgical pain, inflammation, and swelling	
		Treats urinary tract obstructions	
		Helps prevent corneal scars	
		May be helpful with insect and jellyfish stings	
		Accelerates wound healing	
Pectinase	Carbohydrate-digesting	Breaks down carbohydrates, including the fiber pectin found in many fruits and vegetables	Apple juice depectinizing units (AJDUs)
Phytase	Carbohydrate-digesting	Breaks down carbohydrates, particularly phytic acid in the leaves of plants Aids mineral absorption, including iron, calcium, magnesium, and zinc May contain other enzymes, including cellulose and pectinase	Phytase units (PUs)
Protease	Protein-digesting (used as a category of protein-digestive enzymes that includes bromelain, chymotrypsin, papain, pancreatin, and trypsin)	Breaks down protein Supports immune system functioning when taken on an empty stomach Reduces inflammation and increases circulation Aids healing of sports injuries, surgery, wounds Used in chronic conditions like arthritis and cancer	Hemoglobin units in a tyrosine base (HUTs)

Seaprose	Protein-digesting	Breaks down mucus Aids congestion and sinus infections A concentrated form of mucolase	Milligrams (mg)
Serratiopeptidase or serrapeptase or serrapeptidase	Protein-digesting	Breaks down proteins Anti-inflammatory Stimulates immune system Used to treat arthritis, atherosclerosis, fibrocystic breast disease, carpal tunnel syndrome, sinusitis, bronchitis, allergies, psoriasis, ulcerative colitis, multiple sclerosis, cancer; lung secretions Aids in the treatment of injuries, including sprains, strains, torn ligaments Aids antibiotics in treatment of infections	Serratiopeptidase units (SUs) or serrapeptase units or serrapeptidase units
Superoxide dismutase (SOD)	Protein-digesting	Antioxidant that protects the body against free radical damage Anti-inflammatory Treats cataracts Treats temporomandibular joint dysfunction (TMJ) syndrome One of the most potent antioxidant enzymes Requires minerals copper and zinc to function	Milligrams (mg)
Trypsin	Protein-digesting	Breaks down proteins Aids pancreatic insufficiency, intestinal obstructions Aids removal of dead tissue and foreign matter from wounds, ulcerations, fistulas, hematomas, abscesses	Milligrams (mg) or United States Pharmacopeia (USP)

Continued on page 68

Continued from page 67

Common Enzymes and Their Functions[32,33]

Enzyme	Type	Function and Properties	Unit of Measure
		Supports therapy for meningitis	
		Anti-inflammatory	
		Aids hives, scars, dermatitis	
		Treats circulatory disorders	
		Assists surgical repair; reduces postoperative swelling	
		Speeds healing of injuries, including sprains, strains, contusions, factures, black eyes, bruises, tendonitis, bursitis	
		Treats arthritis, gout	
		Treats skin disorders including dermatitis and eczema	
		Aids respiratory and throat conditions, including influenza, bronchitis, lung abscesses, asthma, sinusitis, emphysema, viral pneumonia	
		Treats infections of the urinary tract	
		Helps treat glaucoma and other eye conditions	
		Diabetes: to prevent infected leg ulcers, etc.	
		Helps fight cancer	
Xylanase	Carbohydrate-digesting	A type of hemicellulase that breaks down soluble fiber	Xylanase units (XUs)

Nutrients Required for Enzymes to Work

Eating foods rich in enzymes or popping enzyme supplements is not enough to ensure you'll benefit from their healing abilities. Many nutrients are required to activate enzymes or to function as assistants (called coenzymes). Since our bodies cannot manufacture these nutrients or coenzymes, we must obtain them in our diet.

Minerals

Two minerals, magnesium and zinc, are essential to your body's enzyme health. Magnesium is involved in producing energy that powers most of your bodily processes. You need enough of this important mineral for your body to produce approximately five hundred enzymes that are essential to basic life and metabolism. Magnesium is also involved with vitamin B1 in its many important functions as a coenzyme. Yet some experts estimate that 80 percent of the population is deficient in this mineral. Alfalfa sprouts, almonds, apples, brown rice, celery, dark leafy greens, figs, lemons, sesame seeds, and sunflower seeds are all excellent sources of magnesium.

Zinc is involved in at least three hundred enzyme activities in your body, particularly those that involve the metabolism of carbohydrates (including grains, fruits, sugar, alcohol, and vegetables) and fats. It also supports the pancreatic enzymes, many of which cannot function without it. Zinc too plays an important role in the functioning of one of the most powerful antioxidant enzymes that the body uses to defend itself against disease-causing free radicals—superoxide dismutase (or SOD as it is also known). SOD is one of your body's greatest weapons against aging and disease. To get zinc in your diet, eat beets and beet greens, carrots, green leafy vegetables, nuts, onions, peas, pumpkin seeds, and most types of sprouts.

Coenzymes

Coenzymes include various nutrients, including vitamins B1 and B2, niacin, pantothenic acid, vitamin B6, folate, vitamin B12, biotin, vitamin C, and lipoic acid (also known as coenzyme Q10 or ubiquinone). Our bodies use up coenzymes for important functions and to enable enzymes to work. That means that we need to replace them regularly or we risk depleting our supply of coenzymes, which prevents enzymes from functioning properly.

The first eight nutrients I mentioned above are all part of the B-complex vitamins, so you can see how important it is to ensure that your body has enough B-complex vitamins. All nutrients that function as coenzymes are water soluble and absorbed through the walls of the intestines, where the majority are stored in a form that is bound to enzymes. They play a critical role in a wide variety of biochemical reactions, including cellular energy production. That's part of the reason why so many people who begin to eat a diet rich in B-complex vitamins, or supplement with them alongside a healthy diet, notice an improvement in their energy levels.

Even if you have sufficient enzymes in your body, most of them cannot perform properly without the presence of these important nutrients on an ongoing basis. What's more, in the case of the B-complex vitamins, they are all interdependent and water soluble. That means that if you are deficient in one, you may develop deficiencies in the others as well. And because they are water soluble, they aren't stored in your body, so you must obtain all of them in sufficient quantities on a daily basis. That can be tricky for even the healthiest eaters. Fortunately, a good-quality multivitamin and mineral supplement with high amounts of all the B-vitamins can help, particularly if it is accompanied by improvements in digestion to ensure nutrient absorption.

I've included below a handy chart to help you understand the important role of the B-complex vitamins and their role as coenzymes in your body.

B-Complex Vitamins Function as Coenzymes[34]		
B-Complex Vitamin	**Coenzyme Counterpart or Derivative**	**Primary Function as a Coenzyme**
Vitamin B1 (thiamine)	Thiamine pyrophosphate (TPP)	Energy creation and metabolism
Vitamin B2 (riboflavin)	Flavin mononucleotide (FMN) and flavin adenine dinucleotide (FAD)	Energy creation and metabolism
Niacin (B3)	Nicotinamide adenine dinucleotide (NAD) and Nicotinamide adenine dinucleotide (NADP)	Energy creation and metabolism
Pantothenic Acid (B5)	Coenzyme A and numerous other coenzymes	Energy creation and metabolism
Vitamin B6	Pyridoxal phosphate (PLP) and pyridoxamine phosphate (PMP)	Digestion and absorption of fatty acids found in fats, and amino acids found in protein foods
Folate (B9)	Dihydrofolate (DHF) and tetrahydrofolate (THF)	DNA synthesis
Vitamin B12	Methylcobalamin and deoxyadenosylcobalamin	New cell synthesis and the reformation of folate coenzymes in the body
Biotin	Coenzyme R	Energy creation and metabolism Digestion and absorption of fatty acids from fats, and amino acids from protein foods Synthesis of glycogen (a form of stored energy in the body)

Now that we've explored the amazing healing abilities of enzymes, let's get to work creating the conditions in our bodies that will enable them to have the greatest benefit. In the next chapter, we'll set the stage for enzymes to work their magic. And in Part Two of this book, I'll share specific protocols that I use in my practice to help heal specific health conditions and illnesses.

Setting the Stage for the Phytozyme Cure

Symptoms, then, are in reality nothing but the cry from suffering organs.
—Jean Martin Charcot

Every day, my clients ask me for a natural remedy, nutritional supplement, herb, or homeopathic medicine to alleviate a particular symptom or condition. They want something to relieve pain, alleviate indigestion, or lower high cholesterol. And almost in the same breath, they assure me that they "believe" in holistic medicine. Yet these statements are contradictory. Before I explain why, let me first assure you that "believing" in natural medicine is unnecessary.

The Case for Natural Medicines

Anyone who tells you that there is "no proof" for natural medicines simply hasn't been doing his or her research. Thousands of scientific studies prove the effectiveness of natural medicine. I spend hours every day poring over natural medicine research in scientific journals and databases.

Think about it: Your existence on this planet is proof of the effectiveness of natural medicines. Your ancestors survived thousands of years before pharmaceuticals were invented. They couldn't run to the pharmacy to buy some aspirin for their headaches. Instead they would find some bark of a willow tree or search for the herb meadowsweet, brew it into a tea, and obtain natural salicylic acid to ease their headache pain. Even pharmaceutical giants know the value of natural medicines, since they rely on them as the source for an estimated 75 percent of their drugs. Without effective natural medicine, the human species would have died out long ago. Based on natural medicine's many-thousand-year-old history, along with thousands of modern scientific studies, we know it works.

By comparison, "drug therapy," as most pharmaceutical giants have taken to calling Western medicine, is only a couple hundred years old. It's an infant compared to the wise elder of natural medicine. When you consider the short history of modern drugs in relation to natural medicine's long history, drug-based medicine seems relatively experimental.

In pharmaceutical-based medicine, we go to a doctor, tell the doctor about our symptoms, and ask for a prescription drug to make us feel better. Most people take the same approach to natural medicines. We can't help it—it's an integral part of our way of life and worldview. I call it our "fast-food fix." We want relief, and we want it now.

But taking this approach with your health robs you of the healing potential of a massive, multifaceted, and effective system of medicine that goes deeper than drug therapy. Natural medicine aims to heal the underlying problems causing your symptoms, not just provide a fast symptom fix.

Addressing the Causes of Illness

Consider Sharon as an example. She has a cough and difficulty breathing. She visits her medical doctor and is diagnosed with bronchitis, an inflammation of the bronchial tubes. Her doctor prescribes the following drugs: an albuterol-based inhaler to open her lungs, a corticosteroid to reduce inflammation, and acetaminophen for her fever. The doctor also prescribes an antibiotic to kill bacteria, (although bronchitis is more likely linked to a viral infection, and antibiotics are ineffective against viruses). She takes the prescriptions, and within hours or days her symptoms improve.

Although drugs temporarily made Sharon feel better, they only masked the real problem, and she remained vulnerable to repeated future infections. And so the real question—the one that natural medicine poses—is why did Sharon have bronchitis in the first place?

Like most people, Sharon cursed that nasty little virus she picked up from a friend, family member, or colleague. But Sharon, like everyone, is constantly exposed to countless viruses and other microbes, and yet she's not sick every day. The doctor's diagnosis of "bronchitis" does not say *why* she is sick, only that she *is* sick.

In natural medicine, it is important to determine why a person is experiencing inflammation, why her body was vulnerable to infection at the time, and what led to the weakness in her lungs. Symptoms are clues, not just things to get rid of. In Sharon's case, she had been under a lot of stress at work and home, which overwhelmed her stress glands. She had neglected her normally healthy diet by eating immune system–suppressing sweets (we'll talk more about that later) and lots of highly acid-forming foods like meat (viruses thrive in acidity), and she wasn't getting enough oxygen into her blood through exercise (oxygen helps to kill viruses). Of course, in someone else's situation, the bronchitis may have been linked to any of these factors or a number of other ones. Everyone is different, so slapping a name on a collection of symptoms, and then slapping a grocery list of prescriptions on the condition like a Band-Aid just doesn't cut it. The drug approach may have its merits, but getting to the root cause of the problem is more important.

When symptoms are alleviated through drugs, without adequately assessing a person to learn about the body and its vulnerabilities, it is actually a lost opportunity. That is why there is tremendous wisdom in this chapter's opening quotation from Jean Martin Charcot: "Symptoms, then, are in reality nothing but the cry from suffering organs." So, what happens if you eliminate the symptom, but miss the cry of suffering that your body is trying to communicate to you? The weakness or vulnerability simply shows up again later, and the problem itself is never addressed or solved.

Healing the Whole You

The late pioneering neurosurgeon Harvey Cushing once stated that "a physician is obligated to consider more than a diseased organ, more even than the whole man—he must view the man in his world." A prescription for medicines does not accomplish this. But the skilled health practitioner knows that the cause of disease lies in the lifestyle, habits, mindset, emotions, and diet of the person who is ill.

"Holistic" as in "holistic medicine" concerns itself with the whole person, not just his or her collection of symptoms. One of the tenets of *The Phytozyme Cure* is that your body, even if it is failing in some way or is the source of much discomfort, is actually your ally and not your enemy. When your health fails, it is easy to view your body or a microbe as the problem. But, as my hundreds of clients and thousands of readers can attest, when you give your body what it needs to rebalance, its extraordinary healing powers will do what they need to do.

What Is Phytozyme Therapy?

Throughout this chapter, we're going to discuss ways to set the stage for healing, so that your body is in the best condition possible to receive the benefits of Phytozyme Therapy. Over the last two decades, I've been asking, "What does the body need to achieve balance and well-being?" I've concluded that sometimes what the body needs is as important as what it doesn't need. For example, drinking plenty of pure water is important for the health and well-being of every cell in your body (later in this chapter, I tell you more about how essential it is to get enough water). But if you're drinking primarily cola, replete with colors, sugar (or artificial sweeteners), and preservatives, you need to address both the lack of water and the addition of health-defeating substances to your body.

Your health depends on many factors: oxygen-rich air, plentiful amounts of nutrients, and fresh water, to name a few. While the main factors are the same for everyone, different people do have different requirements. One person may need only 6 cups of water daily, while another may require 10, for example. That's why I've created the Phytozyme Cure to be tailored to your unique health needs.

As we'll explore further in Chapter 4, the three main aspects of the Phtyozyme Cure include:

1. An individualized dietary program tailored to address specific enzyme weaknesses.
2. The use of specific enzymes to remove the barriers to health, including inflammation, pathogens (viruses, bacteria, fungi, and other microbes), and cancer cells.
3. The addition of specific phytonutrient-rich foods and phytonutrient supplements (and other natural remedies) that dramatically bolster the body's healing abilities to speed or increase one's own healing abilities.

In my experience, the potent combination of these three factors can speed and improve healing dramatically, as well as improve a person's health. But if your diet is full of health-harming ingredients, you have a bowel flora imbalance, are suffering from nutritional deficiencies, or you have poor digestion, addressing these concerns first is important, otherwise many of your efforts will be wasted.

Setting the Stage for the Phytozyme Cure

In this chapter, we're going to work on the four main ways to prepare your body for deeper healing. My research and clinical experience show that by working on four main aspects of health, you set the stage for healing. Here's what you need to do:

1. Clean up your diet.
2. Rebalance the bacteria in your body.
3. Supplement with essential vitamins and minerals to address deficiencies and ensure your body has the nutrients required to make adequate enzymes.
4. Improve digestion so your body can absorb the most nutrients possible and defend itself from toxins.

1. Cleaning Up Your Diet

The first step in preparing to feel great is to get rid of the junk that impedes health and may even contribute to illness and disease.

Get the Junk Out

Start by cutting back or (better yet!) eliminating the following substances:

- *Alcohol, tobacco, recreational drugs.* Of course, continue to use any prescription drugs your doctor has recommended.
- *Dairy.* That means milk, cheese, yogurt, sour cream, butter, buttermilk, etc. Many people are sensitive to dairy products but don't know it. Symptoms may be digestive difficulties, bloating, cramping, seasonal allergies, joint or muscle pain, arthritis, among many other symptoms and disorders.
- *Fried foods.* The oils used in fried foods have been heated to temperatures that render the fat rancid and health damaging. Even the healthiest fat when overheated becomes an inflammatory substance that aggravates tissues in the body, including the brain.
- *Sugar, synthetic sweeteners, and sugar substitutes.* Sugar substitutes are worse than their sugary counterparts. They are chemicals that your body was never designed to handle and they are linked

to a whole host of problems: headaches, anxiety attacks, and much more (see the following box, "The Not-So-Sweet Effects of Aspartame" to learn more). If you're craving sweets, start by eating a piece of fruit or drink herbal tea sweetened with stevia (a natural sweetener that does not impact blood sugar levels) or a small amount of raw honey or real maple syrup—no more than 1 teaspoon at a time. Don't confuse stevia, an herb that is naturally sweet, with Splenda, which is not one of the healthy sweeteners that are part of the Phytozyme Cure.

The Not-So-Sweet Effects of Aspartame

I recommend avoiding aspartame because it is a well-documented excitotoxin. An excitotoxin is a substance that literally excites brain or nervous system cells until they die. Research links aspartame to the following health conditions: anxiety attacks; appetite problems such as binge-eating and sugar cravings; birth defects; blindness and vision problems such as blurred vision, bright flashes, and tunnel vision; brain tumors; chest pain; depression and emotional problems; dizziness and vertigo; edema; epilepsy and seizures; fatigue; headaches and migraines; hearing loss and tinnitus; heart palpitations and arrhythmia; hyperactivity; insomnia; joint pain; learning disabilities; memory loss; menstrual irregularities and PMS (premenstrual syndrome); muscle cramps; nausea; numbness of extremities; psychiatric disorders; reproductive problems; skin lesions; slurred speech; and uterine tumors. In extreme cases, aspartame can lead to death.

Aspartame's effects can even be mistaken for Alzheimer's disease, chronic fatigue syndrome, epilepsy, Epstein-Barr virus, Huntington's chorea, hypothyroidism, Lou Gehrig's disease; Lyme disease, Ménière's disease, multiple sclerosis, and post-polio syndrome.[1] Recently, aspartame has had a name change. Now also called "AminoSweet," it is still linked with the same health problems.

Hidden Sources of Sugar

You can find sugar in many unexpected places.[2] Always read labels on any packaged foods before you buy them. If you see any ingredient that ends in "-ose," such as fructose, glucose, maltose, and high fructose corn syrup, know it is actually a form of sugar. As you think about reducing your sugar intake, consider the following ways sugar can sneak into your diet:

- Many meat packers feed sugar to animals prior to slaughter. This improves the flavor and color of cured meat.
- Sugar (in the form of corn syrup and dehydrated molasses) is often added to hamburgers sold in restaurants to reduce shrinkage when the meat is cooked.
- The breading on many prepared foods contains sugar.
- Before salmon is canned, it is often glazed with a sugar solution.
- Some fast-food restaurants sell poultry that has been injected with a honey or sugar solution.
- Sugar is used in the processing of luncheon meats, bacon, and canned meats.
- Such unlikely items as bouillon cubes and dry-roasted nuts have sugar in them.
- Beer, wine, and other alcoholic beverages contain sugar. Champagne and cordials have very high sugar contents.
- Peanut butter and many dry cereals (even corn flakes) contain sugar.
- Some salt contains sugar.
- Almost half the calories found in most commercial ketchups come from sugar.
- Over 90 percent of the calories found in the average can of cranberry sauce come from sugar.

Make Better Choices for a Healthier You

Making healthy food choices is easier than you think. And I guarantee that once you start, you'll begin to feel lighter, more energetic, and clearer mentally, all of which give you greater motivation to eat well. Try these simple steps to a better diet:

- Choose only organic meat and eggs as much as possible. That way, you'll avoid ingesting the growth hormones, estrogens, antibiotics, and other medications that are found in their non-organic counterparts.
- Avoid what I call the "3 Ps"—processed, packaged, and prepared foods. Instead, eat simple homemade meals from fresh ingredients. By eliminating or reducing these foods, you'll automatically be lessening your exposure to preservatives, additives, colors, artificial flavors, and trans fats.
- Choose whole grains over white or wheat products (that includes foods made with white or whole-wheat flour). Instead eat brown rice, millet, oatmeal (not the packaged variety with sweeteners and salt—add 1/2 teaspoon of pure maple syrup and organic cinnamon to taste for a delicious treat), wild rice, and other whole grains I list in the dietary suggestions in Chapter 4 of this book.
- Remember that, contrary to common advice, margarine is not a health food; it is a chemically altered oil that your body was never designed to handle. Instead of margarine, cook with a small amount of olive oil. Or butter your toast with a small amount of coconut oil.
- Switch to Celtic sea salt or Himalayan crystal salt instead of iodized table salt. Or choose another type that contains naturally found minerals alongside the sodium. Usually they have a grayish or slightly orange color due to the minerals present. Of course, if you're a heavy salt user, try to reduce the amount of salt you use.

- Reduce your consumption of coffee or tea to a cup or two a day. (Unless I recommend that you eliminate caffeine altogether because of your specific health concern, which you can determine in Part Two of this book.) Try drinking herbal or green tea instead. Green tea contains some caffeine, but it is substantially less than that in coffee. What's more, green tea is packed with potent healing phytonutrients, and is delicious sweetened with stevia.

- Increase the amount of fiber in your diet. This important step is an easy one, because with the Phytozyme Cure, you'll be eating more vegetables, whole grains, beans, and a small amount of fruit. Most people who eat this way find that their bowel movements become more regular and that they hardly need to give fiber much consideration, since they are naturally consuming more of it.

MSG: The Harmful Hidden Chemical

Many processed, prepared, or packaged foods—the "3 Ps"—contain synthetic ingredients that are linked with many serious health concerns. Many of these synthetic ingredients are known neurotoxins, meaning they are toxins that damage the nervous system or brain. Excitotoxins are a type of neurotoxin. When brain or nerve cells in the body are exposed to excitotoxins, they become excessively excited and fire impulses rapidly until they reach a state of extreme exhaustion. Several hours afterward the brain or nerve cells suddenly die from being excited to death. The effect of literally exciting healthy brain or nerve cells until they die prompted the name neuroscientists gave to these chemicals.

Health Effects of MSG   One of the most readily used neurotoxins is monosodium glutamate, or MSG. Research links MSG to headaches and migraines, hormonal imbalances, hives, mouth eruptions, swelling of mucous membranes (in the oral, gastrointestinal, and reproductive tracts), runny nose, insomnia, seizures, mood swings, panic attacks, diarrhea, heart palpitations and other cardiac irregularities, nausea, numbness, burning, tingling, chest pain, and asthma attacks. If you ever think that MSG is okay in small amounts, it isn't. Research links MSG consumption, even in small doses, to brain and nerve cell death.[3]

MSG has also been linked to excess weight and obesity. In a book by John Erb, a research scientist at the University of Waterloo, called *The Slow Poisoning of America,* he sought to determine how scientists could study obese rats in various experiments, since no rats are naturally obese. He found that when scientists injected rats with MSG when they were first born, their pancreatic output of insulin tripled, resulting in obesity. One recent study of elderly people showed that people eat more when MSG has been added to the food.

Foods That Contain MSG While most people think it is only found in Chinese food, they might be surprised to learn that MSG is commonly used in restaurants and can be found in many processed and prepackaged foods, including canned and boxed soups, dried soup mixes, frozen prepared meals, canned prepared meals, fast food, junk food, snack food, gravy, stew, chili, canned beans, salad dressing, seasoning blends and mixes, bouillon powder and broth, and prepared pasta products.

MSG has been added in larger and larger doses to snacks, fast foods, and even many packaged "health foods." I wish avoiding MSG could be as simple as reading food labels, but MSG often hides in many ingredients, including hydrolyzed vegetable protein, hydrolyzed protein, hydrolyzed plant protein, plant protein extract, sodium caseinate, calcium caseinate, yeast extract, textured vegetable protein (TVP), textured protein, autolyzed yeast, hydrolyzed oat flour, and corn oil. It can be found in flavors added to many foods, often labeled as "natural flavor," "natural beef or chicken flavoring," or "natural flavoring."[4] Soup is one of the most common places you'll find MSG lurking, since bouillon, broth, and stock frequently contains MSG.

Unfortunately, according to Dr. Russell Blaylock, a prominent neurologist and author of *Excitotoxins: The Taste That Kills,* even foods like Chef Boyardee's canned ABC's & 123's that are often marketed to children contain MSG.[5] Children's brains are more susceptible to damage from neurotoxins like MSG, so this is particularly disconcerting.

Knowing all the possible sources of MSG might make you hesitant to eat food that you haven't prepared yourself. It is possible, however, to eat out and still avoid MSG. Many higher quality restaurants that serve only fresh food, cooked from scratch, without bottled sauces and seasonings, are valid options. But, preparing food at home with whole-food ingredients is the best way to avoid it (provided you don't cook with most bottled sauces, spice mixtures, and flavorings).

Lessening the Damage from MSG There are specific nutrients that can counteract some of the damage from MSG, but knowing this is not an excuse to eat more junk foods that contain this harmful neurotoxin. It is valuable to know the ways to minimize MSG's possible damaging effects because it is difficult to avoid it all of the time, particularly when eating out or traveling.

Dr. Blaylock cites research in his book *Excitotoxins* that demonstrates that vitamin E has been shown to significantly block the toxic effect of glutamate in brain cells.[6] He also indicates that magnesium and moderate doses of zinc (25 to 50 milligrams daily) can lessen the toxic effects of MSG.[7] Research published in the journal *Phytomedicine* indicated that a combination of nutrients found in the herb red clover mitigated some of the damage from MSG for participants of the study. Another study in *Phytomedicine* found that standardized extracts of the herb Saint-John's-wort was also helpful.

Just remember that you should not use these nutrients and herbs as an excuse to eat anything you want. Because no food or herb has been proven to completely prevent damaging health effects of eating foods containing MSG, it is still important to avoid it as much as possible.

2. Having the Guts to Be Healthy—Balancing Bacteria

As you learned in Chapter 2, your intestines are home to many microorganisms—somewhere in the 100 trillion range. Most of these bacteria are beneficial, actually essential, to the formation of nutrients like vitamin B12 as well as to the manufacture of approximately three thousand enzymes in your body. However, some can be pathogenic and have a disruptive effective on health and well-being. Provided the body can keep the ratio of healthy microbes to pathogenic ones to a ratio of about 85:15, you will experience intestinal health (and probably overall health as well). However, for many people the balance can tip in favor of the harmful pathogens, which is called dysbiosis.

There are many reasons dysbiosis can occur, including excess sugar intake, alcohol consumption, birth control pill use, antibiotic use, stress, an imbalanced body chemistry, insufficient dietary fiber, not drinking enough water, and more.

A particular yeast called *Candida albicans* has an affinity for the intestines and can become overgrown there. This yeast can release over 80 known toxins and create a pH imbalance that makes it difficult for your body to manufacture the enzymes it needs to function properly. These toxins can also cause the mucous membranes of the intestines to become damaged and leaky, allowing undigested protein molecules or toxins to be absorbed into the bloodstream.

Causes of Harmful Bacteria or Candida Overgrowth

- Alcohol intake (wine, beer, champagne, hard liquor, etc.)
- Antibiotic use
- Birth control pills
- Blood sugar imbalances

- Consumption of foods that contain antibiotics and hormones (meat, poultry, dairy products)
- Excessive sugar, bread, or wheat consumption
- Immunosuppressive drug use (steroids, cortisone, etc.)
- Mercury amalgam dental fillings
- Sex with an infected partner
- Nutritional deficiencies
- Poor diet
- Recreational drug use
- Smoking
- Stress
- Toxic exposures, especially to mold
- Weakened immunity

Research shows that the yeast candida can stimulate histamine production, causing excessive allergies. It can also produce hormone-like substances that interfere with the body's own hormone balance. And as you can see from the following "Do You Have Yeast Overgrowth?" quiz, candida can be linked to many other health conditions. So it is important to get on top of it early in any health program.

Do You Have Yeast Overgrowth?

There are many symptoms of yeast overgrowth. Do you suffer from the following symptoms or conditions?

- Acne, psoriasis, eczema, rashes, or hives
- Allergies
- Anal, vaginal, or jock itch
- Anemia
- Anxiety
- Asthma

- Athlete's foot
- Attention-deficit/hyperactivity disorder (ADHD) or attention deficit disorder (ADD)
- Autism
- Bloating and flatulence
- Body odor or bad breath
- Brain fog or memory lapses
- Chemical sensitivities
- Constipation or diarrhea
- Cravings for sweets, bread, or alcohol
- Crohn's disease
- Depression
- Difficulty gaining or losing weight
- Diminished libido
- Fatigue that sleep doesn't help
- Fibromyalgia
- Food sensitivities
- Headaches, especially frequent
- Heartburn
- Hormonal imbalances
- Hypoglycemia
- Immune dysfunction
- Indecisiveness
- Insomnia
- Irritable bowel syndrome
- Joint or muscle aches
- Lack of concentration
- Mood swings or irritability
- Nasal congestion
- Premenstrual syndrome
- Recurrent bladder, sinus, vaginal yeast, or respiratory infections
- Thyroid conditions
- Unexplained weight changes

If you experience some or many of these symptoms or conditions, you may need to address candida overgrowth as part of the Phytozyme Cure. Cleaning up your diet based on the earlier suggestions, combined with eating more phytonutrient-rich food and supplementing with enzymes, goes a long way toward eliminating a candida overgrowth. However, sometimes you need to take additional steps. Always consult your doctor to rule out any serious medical conditions that may be causing the above symptoms.

Steady Your Blood Sugar Levels

There are numerous ways to address a bacterial imbalance or yeast overgrowth in the intestines.

First, it is important to eliminate the contributing factors as much as possible. Quit smoking and recreational drug use, reduce alcohol intake, and minimize consumption of sugar and sugary foods, wheat and white bread.

One of the tenets of the Phytozyme Cure is the necessity to balance blood sugar levels. Balanced blood sugar levels are critical to good health, stable energy levels, and maintaining a healthy weight. When our blood sugar levels drop, we feel hungry and are likely to eat. When we eat something sweet, our blood sugar spikes, causing the pancreas to secrete insulin in response. Eating something sweet tends to cause glucose levels to become too high. In response, the body converts the excess glucose to glycogen (a short-term fuel stored mainly in the liver and muscle cells) or fat, our long-term energy reserve. Within an hour or so, blood sugar drops dramatically, causing us to crave sweets or something sugary to restore blood sugar levels. If our blood sugar levels become too low we may experience fatigue, poor concentration, irritability, nervousness, depression, headaches, sweating, or digestive difficulties. It can become a vicious cycle. Eating sporadically is just as problematic. When we skip meals or leave more than two to three hours between eating, our blood sugar drops dramatically, causing many of the same problems.

Incidentally, for those who are overweight or would like to lose weight, keep in mind that blood sugar fluctuations can cause the body to hoard fat by mistakenly thinking it may be starving. Blood sugar imbalances can also worsen many of the symptoms for most health problems. If excess glucose continues over long periods of time, obesity may result. Diabetes may result when the body no longer produces sufficient insulin (the hormone that carries glucose from the blood to the cells). Maintaining balanced blood sugar may be the single most important factor to maintain energy levels, balance weight, experience good health, and prevent illnesses like diabetes.

Eat Regularly

So it is important to stabilize blood sugar. One of the easiest ways to do so is to eat every two to three hours and to avoid sugary foods and the "white" foods like white flour, white sugar, white potatoes, and white rice.

Another easy way to stabilize blood sugar is to keep snacks containing protein and fiber handy to eat every couple of hours. That could include celery with almond butter, or a handful of unsalted raw almonds, cashews, or sunflower seeds. Eating protein with every meal is also important to address bacterial or candida overgrowth. While protein can come from wild fish or organic chicken, turkey, eggs, or lean beef, it need not be meat. You can also eat beans and lentils, nuts and nut butter, seeds, sprouts, or other vegetarian sources of protein.

Supplement with Probiotics

Supplement your diet with a high-quality probiotic, preferably one containing a wide variety of bacterial strains. The one I use contains *Streptococcus thermophilus, Propionibacterium freudenreichii, Lactobacillus rhamnosus, Lactobacillus plantarum, Lactobacillus paracasei, Lactobacillus bulgaricus, Lactobacillus acidophilus, Bifidobacterium longum, Bifidobacterium lactis, Bifidobacterium infantis, Bifidobacterium breve,*

Bifidobacterium bifidum. Don't worry about remembering their lengthy names. I added the information here so you could take this book with you when you go shopping at your local health food store. Usually the word "Lactobacillus" will be shortened to "L." and "Bifidobacterium" will be shortened to "B." on product labels.

Usually bacteria are measured in colony forming units—(CFU) for short—and most types will have between 1 and 20 billion CFU. Or the package may just indicate, say, 4 billion per capsule. However, don't be fooled into thinking that choosing a quality probiotic is just a numbers game. I recently overheard a man in my local health food store telling the clerk that he wanted the probiotic with the greatest variety of bacteria strains and the highest number of bacteria per capsule. The product she gave him was one that I am familiar with and, while it came with the highest price tag, was definitely not the best-quality product.

So how do you choose a good-quality probiotic? Well, give the numbers some consideration, but there are two true tests of a good probiotic: (1) it has a beneficial impact on your body (most people will know within a day to two weeks), or (2) it will turn milk (or soy milk) into yogurt.

It is important to take probiotic supplements on an empty stomach and away from antibiotics or oregano oil supplements. I find the ideal time is either before bed or first thing in the morning. If you take it in the morning, try to leave at least 20 to 30 minutes before eating.

Another way to rebalance your intestinal bacteria is by eating fermented foods like sauerkraut, yogurt, and miso (fermented soy).

People often ask me, "Can't I just eat yogurt instead of taking a probiotic supplement?" Yes, you can. But if you have a severe bacterial or yeast infection, you may need probiotic supplements, which tend to be stronger and more effective.

Choose Antibacterial Herbs

Depending on the number of symptoms you have and the severity of the possible bacterial imbalance, you may also need to choose anti-parasitic foods and herbs to kill harmful ones. Some of the best ones include garlic, onions, scallions, horseradish (preservative- and dairy-free types), ginger, and oregano oil. If you're supplementing with oregano oil, be sure to take it two to three hours before or after your probiotic supplement, since it indiscriminately kills intestinal bacteria quite effectively.

You may also benefit from following the suggestions listed under "Yeast Infections" in Part Two of this book.

3. Addressing Nutrient Deficiencies

While I truly believe food is the best medicine, today's food supply is deficient in many essential nutrients. And, let's face it: few people are eating the perfect diet. So it is important to add a good-quality vitamin and mineral supplement to address possible deficiencies.

For many people, a multivitamin and mineral supplement along with a healthy diet and improved digestion will address possible nutrient deficiencies. However, if you are suffering from a long-standing or serious health condition, experience a large amount of stress, eat a poor diet, drink alcohol, smoke, don't get sufficient exercise, or exercise a lot, it may no longer be adequate. Chronic illness also places extra nutritional demands on your body and may even be the result of, at least in part, nutritional deficiencies.

And, these nutrient deficiencies can be the result of enzyme deficiencies. In Part Two, I encourage you to start taking a full-spectrum digestive enzyme along with every meal and snack. Start now and take it alongside your multivitamin and mineral to assist with absorbing the nutrients in the supplement and in the food you're eating.

Some people need more vitamins or minerals than a multivitamin provides. To help you figure out if you need additional supplementation, I have compiled some charts of deficiency symptoms. The charts are intended only as guidelines. Some of the symptoms are fairly general and may be symptoms of other health conditions as well. There are many more vitamins and minerals than those indicated in the charts, so it is always a good idea to work with a skilled nutritional medicine practitioner who can help you address any potential deficiencies. I also make condition-specific vitamin and mineral supplementation recommendations in Part Two to help you select the ones that may be beneficial for you.

Vitamin A

Vitamin A is an important antioxidant vitamin that helps neutralize free radicals in your body. Free radicals are linked to aging and disease. Vitamin A also plays a role in healthy hair, nails, skin, eyes, bones, teeth, and adrenal glands (your body's stress glands). Your body can make vitamin A from the phytonutrient beta-carotene, which, as you learned in Chapter 1, is found in carrots, mangoes, melon, papayas, squash, and dark green vegetables. However, if you are diabetic, your body may lack this ability, and it may be essential to obtain vitamin A directly from fish oils or supplementation.

Common Signs and Symptoms of a Vitamin A Deficiency
Acne or blackheads
Cysts or boils in ears or mouth
Dry eyes
Dry hair, split ends, or hair falling out
Dry, scaly, or red eyelids
Dry or scaly skin
Eyes have difficulty adjusting when entering a dark room
Eye inflammation or pink eye (conjunctivitis)
Eyes sensitive to sunlight, glare, or bright lights
Frequent colds, flu, or other infections
Reduced night vision or inability to see in dim light
Rough bumps on the back of arms
Sinus problems or sinusitis
Swollen eyelids or sties on eyelids
Urinary tract infections (including bladder or kidney infections, also called cystitis)
Warts

B-Complex Vitamins

The B-complex vitamins play important roles in your body. Not only do they serve as coenzymes that assist enzymes with their thousands of functions, they are also essential to manufacture hormones, aid with stress management in your body, help balance moods, increase energy, aid reproduction, manage pain and pain signals, heal wounds, assist memory and learning capacity, boost immunity, and help balance glandular functions. There are many vitamins within the complex, including B1, B2, niacin, pantothenic acid, B6, folate, B12, B13, B15, B17, choline, inositol, biotin, and PABA. (Don't worry about trying to remember all of these vitamins, their names, or their critical roles in your body. You can always refer back to this chapter.)

Beans, cantaloupe, citrus fruits, whole grains, kale, pumpkin seeds, brown rice, strawberries, green veggies, and root vegetables are good sources of the B-complex vitamins. Most people experience greater energy and balanced moods soon after eating a diet rich in B-complex vitamins and/or supplementing with them.

Common Signs and Symptoms of a B-Complex Vitamin Deficiency
Abnormal hair loss
Anemia, fatigue, or weakness
Anxiety, irritability, or nervousness
Cold sores or canker sores in mouth
Depression, anxiety, or irritability
Dizzy or light-headed when standing up
Dry hair, split ends, or abnormal hair loss
Fleeting pains or tenderness in joints or legs
Forgetfulness or short attention span
Frequent colds, flu, or other infections
Hangnails, or cuticles tear easily

Continued on page 94

Continued from page 93

Common Signs and Symptoms of a B-Complex Vitamin Deficiency
Headaches
Heart palpitations or slow or rapid heartbeat
High blood pressure
Insomnia or difficulty staying asleep
Irregular heartbeat
Lack of endurance or fatigue easily
Muscle cramps in legs, especially after exercising
Prematurely aging skin or wrinkling
Rapid heartbeat with slightest exertion
Restless leg syndrome
Shortness of breath or chest pains
Skin bruises easily
Skin is itchy, red, or inflamed (dermatitis)
Weight loss or loss of appetite
White skin patches
Women: Acne or swelling is worse during periods; menstrual problems; morning sickness during pregnancy

Vitamin C

Like vitamin A, vitamin C is an antioxidant nutrient that lessens free radical damage linked to disease and aging in the body. It is helpful to boost immunity, form bones and teeth, and aid digestion and blood cell formation. It also helps accelerate wound healing, produces collagen that maintains skin's youthful elasticity, and helps your body cope with stress. Vitamin C is one of the most important nutrients to help your glands manage stress, something most of us take for granted until our energy reserves fail us after severe stress. Rich sources of vitamin C include black currants, beet greens, grapefruit, lemons, limes, oranges, red peppers, pomegranates, spinach, strawberries, tomatoes, and many types of sprouts.

Common Signs and Symptoms of a Vitamin C Deficiency
Anemia
Excessive hair loss
Exhaust easily
Fragile bones
Frequent nosebleeds
Gums bleed easily, especially when brushing or flossing teeth
Premature aging of skin
Prone to catching cold, flu, or other infections
Skin bruises easily
Sores, wounds, or infections heal slowly

Vitamin D

Vitamin D plays essential roles in supporting our energy and balancing our moods. It also helps to build healthy bones, heart, nerves, skin, and teeth, and it supports the health of the thyroid gland—a butterfly-shaped gland in the throat that helps maintain a healthy weight, balanced metabolism, and energy levels.

New evidence shows that people with higher levels of vitamin D experienced a decreased risk of type 2 diabetes. Researchers at the US Department of Agriculture's Human Nutrition Research Center on Aging at Tufts University just released its study linking low levels of vitamin D to diabetes in the *American Journal of Clinical Nutrition*.[8] The authors of the study concluded that maintaining optimal vitamin D levels in the blood may be a type 2 diabetes prevention strategy.

Other recent research found that vitamin D plays a critical role in activating the body's immune system against infectious diseases like the flu.[9] Researchers note that a deficiency in this important vitamin, which actually acts like a hormone in your body, may result in a greater risk of contracting flu viruses. Also, additional research has linked low amounts of vitamin D to autoimmune disorders, cancer, depression, diabetes, and heart disease.[10]

Many people incorrectly think that getting a bit of sunshine daily is sufficient to meet their vitamin D requirements. However, after your skin is exposed to sunlight, it takes about 48 hours to convert it into vitamin D. During that time, the sunlight-initiated precursors to vitamin D can be washed off with soap and water. So, if you scrub your skin with soap in the shower, your body will not convert most of your skin's sun exposure to vitamin D. I'm not suggesting that you avoid showering after sun exposure, rather, that you primarily soap the areas that don't usually see the light of day and wash the sun-exposed ones with water only.

Vitamin D is also found in food such as fish and fish oils, sweet potatoes, sunflower seeds, mushrooms, and many types of sprouts. People with low thyroid function (hypothyroidism) tend to have difficulty with vitamin D absorption and, as a result, tend to have higher needs for this nutrient. For most people I recommend supplementation of 2000 to 4000 IU daily.

Common Signs and Symptoms of a Vitamin D Deficiency
Bow legs or knock-knee (rickets)
Burning in mouth or throat
Constipation
Dental cavities or cracked teeth
Insomnia
Joint pains or bone pains
Muscle cramps
Nearsightedness or myopia (can't see distances)
Nervousness
Osteomalacia
Osteoporosis
Poor bone development

Vitamin E

Like vitamins A and C, vitamin E is an antioxidant vitamin that helps combat the effects of aging and prevent disease. It also supports healthy blood vessels, the heart, liver, lungs, adrenal and pituitary glands, skin, testes, and uterus, as well as other tissues. It also helps to protect your body against food and environmental toxins. It is found in cereals, whole grains and whole-grain breads, and many types of sprouts, as well as in leafy dark green vegetables, nuts, and seeds.

Common Signs or Symptoms of a Vitamin E Deficiency
Anemia
Blood clots or tendency to form blood clots
Celiac disease
Cystic fibrosis
Dry hair, split ends, or hair falling out
Eye twitching
Men: impotence or low sex drive
Muscle weakness or swelling or loss of muscle mass
Poor coordination
Women: menstrual pain

Calcium

Most people equate calcium with bones. From what we currently know about calcium, however, it may be involved with more bodily functions than any other mineral. It is involved in the health of your bones, muscles, and heart, as well as many of your body's cells. While dairy products contain calcium, they are not typically the best source of calcium for most people. Even if you get lots of calcium from dairy products, your body may not be digesting it adequately to extract enough calcium to meet its needs. Although Americans and Canadians tend to consume the highest amount of dairy products in the world per capita, we have a higher incidence of osteoporosis than most other countries. We also suffer from many of the other calcium-deficiency symptoms.

But you don't have to consume dairy to get bone-building benefits. Highly usable sources of calcium include almonds and almond butter, broccoli, carrot juice, dark leafy greens, kale, kelp, navy beans, oats, and sesame seeds and sesame butter (tahini).

Common Signs and Symptoms of a Calcium Deficiency
Back or hip pain
Bone loss, malformed bones, or bones that are vulnerable to fractures or breaks
Brittle nails or vertical ridges on nails
Cramps in feet, toes, or legs
Dental cavities or frequent toothaches
Headaches
Heart palpitations
High blood pressure
Insomnia
Joint pain
Nervousness, anxiety, or irritability
Nervous tics or twitches, or muscles that twitch
Women: painful or lengthy periods or excessive bleeding during periods

Chromium

Chromium helps to maintain a strong heart and healthy artery and blood function. It also helps alleviate cravings for sweets, mood swings, and weight gain linked to fluctuating blood sugar levels. It is intricately linked to energy production in our bodies. Naturally found in sugarcane, this nutrient is removed from the cane when it is refined into white sugar. It is found in potatoes, beans, and many whole grains.

Common Signs and Symptoms of a Chromium Deficiency
Cravings for sugary or starchy foods
Diabetes or hypoglycemia (or chronically high or low blood sugar)
Difficulty tolerating alcohol or sugar
High cholesterol
High triglycerides

Iodine

Iodine's main job is ensuring healthy thyroid gland functioning. The thyroid gland is a butterfly-shaped gland in the throat that aids energy, mood, metabolism, temperature regulation, and balanced weight. Iodine also helps to support the healthy functioning of the brain and nervous system, and is needed for healthy hair, nails, skin, and teeth. While iodine has been added to table salt, I don't recommend table salt as a source of this valuable mineral. Instead, choose seaweed like agar, arame, dulse, kelp, wakame, or other types of seaweed. Garlic, peaches, pears, pineapples, pumpkins, sesame seeds, watercress, zucchini, and Himalayan crystal or Celtic sea salt (use moderately) also contain some iodine.

Common Signs and Symptoms of an Iodine Deficiency
Brittle nails
Cold hands and/or feet
Constipation
Dry hair
Heart palpitations
High cholesterol levels
Irritability
Overweight or obesity
Slow mental reactions
Slow metabolism
Thyroid enlargement or goiter
Women: fibrocystic breasts or breast lumps

Iron

Iron is a key constituent of enzymes that are essential to your immune system's ability to attack foreign invaders such as bacteria, fungi, and viruses. It also plays important roles in red and white blood cell production, your body's ability to cope with stress, proper immune functioning, and metabolism of protein foods. Iron is found in asparagus, apricots, bananas, beans, figs, dark leafy greens, kelp, lentils, peaches, prunes, raisins, red meat, and walnuts. And here's a bonus: the vegetarian sources of iron listed here also contain vitamin C, which aids iron absorption.

Common Signs and Symptoms of an Iron Deficiency
Breathing difficulties
Brittle or soft nails or vertical ridges on nails
Chronic fatigue
Cravings for ice or tendency to eat ice
Intolerance to cold
Lack of stamina or endurance
Nails are flat or concave (curved in like spoons)
Pale fingernails
Pale inner skin on lower eyelid
Pale skin
Poor attention span
Weakened immune system

Magnesium

Magnesium is essential for your body to manufacture over five hundred enzymes that are essential to metabolic functions. It aids sleep, helps combat stress, and is needed for healthy artery, bone, blood, heart, muscle, and nerve functions. Magnesium is vital to health. Even our bodies' genetic material is dependent on adequate supplies of magnesium. Yet experts estimate that approximately 80 percent of North Americans are deficient in this critical nutrient. You can incorporate magnesium into your diet with alfalfa sprouts, almonds, apples, celery, figs, leafy greens, lemons, brown rice, sesame seeds, and sunflower seeds.

Common Signs and Symptoms of a Magnesium Deficiency
Back pain
Carpal tunnel syndrome
Chronic fatigue

Confusion

Cravings for chocolate

Depression

Dizziness

Epilepsy or convulsions

Excessive body odor

Heart palpitations or irregular heartbeat

High blood pressure

Hyperactivity or restlessness

Inability to control bladder

Insomnia

Irritability or anxiety

Muscle cramps or muscle tension

Nervous tics or twitches, or muscles that twitch or spasm

Painful and cold feet or hands

Pain in knees or hips

Restless legs, especially at night

Seizures, convulsions, or tremors

Sensitive or loose teeth

Women: PMS or painful periods

Potassium

Potassium, like calcium, magnesium, and sodium, is one of the electrolyte minerals. Like other electrolytes, potassium performs many essential functions, including relaxing muscles, converting glucose into fuel for the body, reducing swelling, protecting and controlling kidney function, regulating bodily fluids, and balancing acid-alkalinity. (For more information on the latter function, consult my book *The Ultimate pH Solution*.) You need adequate potassium to maintain the health of your heart, kidneys, muscles, nerves, and skin. Good sources of potassium include apricots, bananas, citrus fruits, whole grains, potatoes, sunflower seeds, tomatoes, and most vegetables (especially dark green leafy ones).

Common Signs and Symptoms of a Potassium Deficiency
Constipation
Dry skin
Extreme thirst
Fluid retention in hands or ankles
Heart palpitations, irregular heartbeat, slow or rapid heartbeat
High blood pressure
Irritability or easily agitated
Muscular weakness
Painful or abnormally stiff muscles after exercising

Silica

Important to bone-building, immune system strengthening, the proper use of calcium in the body, and building strong nails, hair, and teeth, silica also supports an enzyme called prolyhydroxylase that is involved in the formation of collagen in bones, cartilage, and connective tissue. Silica is found in almonds, apples, beets, celery, flaxseed, whole grains, grapes, kelp, oats, onions, parsnips, strawberries, and sunflower seeds.

Common Signs and Symptoms of a Silica Deficiency
Excessive wrinkling of the skin
Insomnia
Irritability
Muscle cramps
Poor bone development
Soft or brittle nails
Thinning or loss of hair

Zinc

Zinc is necessary for your body to manufacture over three hundred different enzymes that it needs for life and metabolism. This critical nutrient is necessary for healing burns and wounds, and for properly digesting carbohydrate foods like grains, fruits, and sugars, as well as protein foods like meat, eggs, and beans. Our blood, bones, brain, heart, liver, and muscles depend on adequate levels of this mineral to function properly. Men tend to have higher zinc needs than women, to support healthy prostate functioning. Zinc is found in many types of sprouts, beet greens, beets, carrots, nuts, onions, peas, pumpkin seeds, sunflower seeds, and dark leafy green vegetables.

Common Signs and Symptoms of a Zinc Deficiency
Acne
Anorexia or small appetite
Brittle nails
Children/teenagers: growing pains, stunted growth
Diarrhea
Difficulty conceiving children
Frequent colds, flu, or infections
Hair or nails grow slowly
Loss of sense of smell or taste
Men: late sexual maturity, prostate disorders, impotence, or low sperm count
Sleep disturbances
Slow-healing wounds or injuries
Stretch marks
White spots on fingernails

Drink Up—Getting More Water

We constantly hear about the importance of drinking enough water. On the flip side, recent media reports say that the commonly recommended 8 cups of water daily is a myth, which is technically accurate but not the whole story, because different people require different amounts of water to feel their best and be properly hydrated. Regardless of whether you need 8 cups of water daily, or 4 or 10, most people are not getting the message that whatever their particular water needs are, they aren't meeting them.

And even dietitians, nutritionists, and medical professionals are contributing to the problem by informing people that they get enough water in their diet in the form of fruits and vegetables. That might be true for some people, but after assessing the diets of hundreds of people, I assure you that isn't the case for most.

Plus, have you ever noticed that when you throw vegetables in a pan and turn on the heat, you see liquid in the pan, and then steam? That's because you're literally cooking the water out of the vegetables.

More than two-thirds of your body weight is water. Without adequate water your body's biochemical and electrical (yes, electrical, read on!) processes begin to break down. The list of reasons your body needs water is as plentiful as the functions in your body, but due to space limitations, here are just 11 good reasons to drink more water:

1. Your blood is over 80 percent water and needs water to make healthy new blood cells.

2. Your bones are over 50 percent water and, you guessed it, need water to make healthy new bone cells.

3. Drinking more water helps lessen pain in your body by getting your lymphatic system moving. The lymphatic system is a network of nodes, tubes, vessels, and fluid that moves waste out of your tissues. It requires water to function properly.

4. Water helps to eliminate wastes and toxins from your body through the lymphatic system, kidneys, and intestines.

5. Water lubricates your joints and helps reduce joint pain and protect against wear and tear.

6. Water regulates your metabolism, so if you're overweight, chances are you may need to drink more water.

7. Water balances your body temperature.

8. Water helps to ensure adequate electrical functioning so your brain and nervous system can work. Your brain and nervous system send out electrical signals to function properly.

Researchers estimate that your brain gives off about the same amount of electricity as a 60-watt light bulb. So, there's some truth to the image of a light bulb going on when someone has a good idea.

9. Water alleviates dehydration (and I've already mentioned that most people are chronically dehydrated).

10. As you learned in Chapter 2, your body needs adequate water for enzymes to work properly. That includes your metabolic and digestive enzymes.

11. Every cell and organ in your body requires adequate water to function properly.

One of the quickest and easiest ways to improve your health is to start drinking more pure water every day. Be sure to drink water on an empty stomach or you'll simply be diluting your digestive enzymes and making your digestion less effective.

Choose purified water as much as possible (but get yourself a reusable BPA-free water bottle so you won't pollute your body or the planet with all those plastic water bottles). In wealthy, developed nations with easy access to clean water, we really have no excuse for being dehydrated.

4. Improving Your Digestion

You are what you eat, according to the old adage. But, I think "and you are what you digest and absorb" is an important addition to the saying. After all, what you eat, digest, and absorb will become the building blocks of *every* cell in your body. Great health *requires* great building blocks.

Carbohydrates, fats, and proteins provide the foundation for every single tissue, organ, and organ system in your body, in the form of sugars, essential fats, and amino acids. Without adequate "macronutrients," as these building blocks are also called, your immune system, brain, hormonal systems, detoxification mechanisms, or any other system in the body would not work properly.

For example, if proteins go undigested, you can (1) suffer from an amino acid deficiency, no matter how much protein you eat, and (2) experience a leaky gut, which can lead to a whole host of problems, ranging from allergies to autoimmune disorders like rheumatoid arthritis, lupus, multiple sclerosis, some forms of hypothyroidism, pain disorders, and much more.

Once these toxins or undigested proteins enter the blood, the body attacks them. If they find their way to organs, glands, or tissues, the body may begin to attack these organs, glands, and tissues, which over time can result in serious damage. So you can see why correcting digestive problems and bacterial overgrowth, and ensuring proper digestion of foods is essential to enzyme formation and overall health.

Even if you think your digestion is fine and that you don't need to improve upon it, please keep reading. Strong, healthy digestion really is the foundation upon which great health is built.

Going With, Not Against, Your Gut

Most people have compromised digestion, largely due to poor food and beverage choices. Because we overeat, we are used to experiencing a heavy, bloated feeling. So, even if you think your digestion is perfect, it is imperative to follow the suggestions below. Whether your body has the building blocks of healthy cells, tissues, and organs is largely determined by the power of your digestion, along with your food choices. By now, you should have cleaned up your diet, which goes a long way toward improved digestion and better health.

It need not be difficult to improve your digestion. The overall health results of making a few changes to how, when, and what you eat will astound you. Not only will you have less indigestion, flatulence, constipation, diarrhea, or other digestive difficulties, you'll also find other negative symptoms improve. The reason is simple: you'll absorb more nutrients from your food and fewer waste products into your bloodstream.

7 Easy Ways to Improve Your Digestion

1. Chew, chew, chew your food. Then, chew it some more. As you may recall, enzymes in foods are released by chewing them well. Plus chewing well allows food to mingle longer with your salivary juices, helping to break them down further and ensuring more digestion occurs in the upper chamber of the stomach.

2. Don't drink with meals. Or, if you have supplements to take with meals, drink a small amount of water. Not only does drinking with meals dilute the enzymes in your food and your body's digestive juices, it prematurely raises the pH of your stomach—the signal that tells your stomach to dump stomach contents into the duodenum. That means undigested foods will prematurely find their way to your intestines, where they may cause inflammation or leak through the intestinal walls—a precursor to many illnesses.

3. Simplify your meals. Heavy, complex meals like a steak, baked potato, gravy, cake and ice cream are harder to digest than simpler, lighter ones. Digestion requires a tremendous amount of energy and enzymes. Take the burden off your body by simplifying your diet.

4. Try not to eat when you are stressed out. If you are always stressed, learn some stress-management techniques. You're the only person who can manage the stress in your life. Emotional distress diverts a substantial amount of energy needed for digestion.

5. Eat prior to 7:00 or 7:30 p.m. That gives your body time to digest foods thoroughly before going to bed. If you work night shifts, avoid eating for at least three hours before bed. That means no late-night snacks. It also means you can take a probiotic supplement on an empty stomach before bed (refer back to "Supplement with Probiotics" starting on page 89).

6. Add a full-spectrum digestive enzyme to your meals. (You learned about digestive enzyme supplements in the last chapter. Refer back if you need a quick reminder.)

7. Make sure you are taking a probiotic supplement as I suggest above on a morning and/or nightly basis.

Remember, great digestion is the foundation for great health. By improving your digestion, you'll be making big strides to improve your overall well-being. Your body will thank you in the form of comfortable digestion, more energy, and healthy weight.

By following these ways to set the stage for the Phytozyme Cure, you're preparing to discover your Phytozyme Cure Type, address any enzyme deficiencies you might have, and customize your diet and supplement program to suit your type and health conditions. You're well on your way to experience renewed vitality, increased immunity, and supercharged healing.

4

The Phytozyme Cure

*The only person you are destined to become is
the person you decide to be.*
—Ralph Waldo Emerson

At this point, you've already come a long way in your quest to heal your body. You have a good understanding of phytonutrients and enzymes, and you've made some dietary changes to help get the most out of their healing abilities. Now I'll tell you how to customize your diet (and the enzymes you get from your diet) to suit your individual needs.

In Part Two of this book, you'll find out more about supplementing your diet with the specific phytonutrients and enzymes, and how doing so can work to improve and heal over 30 specific health conditions. But before you do, I'll help you discover your Phytozyme Cure Type[1] by looking at your potential enzyme weaknesses and how you can address them with foods that are best suited to your particular type. Let's get started.

Discovering Your Phytozyme Cure Type

By discovering your Phytozyme Cure Type, you can start eating the right kinds of foods for your body to maximize your genetic potential and start experiencing greater energy, improved resistance to illness, and vibrant good looks. You may recall from Chapter 2 that there are four Phytozyme Cure Types: Carbohydrate, Fat, Protein, and Combination. Your Phytozyme Cure Type reflects likely enzyme deficiencies that you may be experiencing. There are three main reasons for these deficiencies:

1. You don't get enough enzymes in your overall diet.
2. You may be eating more of a particular type of food than your body can handle.
3. You may have an inherent weakness in digesting certain types of food.

Of course, you can easily start eating more enzyme-rich food to help counter the first reason (consult my book *The Life Force Diet* for more information on eating an enzyme-rich diet). The latter two issues can be addressed through shifts in your diet and supplementation with extra enzymes.

What Your Weaknesses Say about You

Let's face it: no one is good at everything. We all have weaknesses. Enzyme weaknesses are no different from skill sets. My sister was an amazing basketball player, but I couldn't efficiently run and dribble a ball if my life depended on it. Running without a basketball was a whole different game—that's where I excelled. Someone who is an expert chef may not be the best novelist. An accountant may not be the best painter. The same is true of enzymes: we all have strengths and we all have weaknesses. While I'd love to focus on the strengths, it really is the weaknesses that determine your level of health. So, your Phytozyme Cure Type identifies your weaknesses—the type of foods that you may have trouble digesting and/or the enzymes with which you need to supplement.

Take the three quizzes in this chapter to help you to determine your Phytozyme Cure Type. Each quiz reflects the main symptoms and conditions that have been linked to deficiencies in the enzymes that digest starches and sugars, fats, and proteins. These enzymes include amylase; sucrase, lactase, and maltase (also sometimes lumped together under the category of disaccharidases); lipase; and protease respectively.

You may notice that there is no Fiber Type. That's because we don't have enzymes in our bodies to digest fibrous foods. That doesn't mean you should avoid foods that contain fiber—fruit, vegetables, grains, nuts, beans, and seeds. These foods are good for us. Remember (from Chapter 2) that in their raw, unadulterated state, these foods contain the enzymes needed to digest them. That includes cellulase (or cellulose as it is also called) to digest fiber.

Consider carbohydrates, or "carbs" as most people called them. Carbs include starchy foods, sugary foods, fruit, and even vegetables, and the fiber they contain. While carbs have gotten a bad rap thanks to the dieting industry, many carbs are beneficial and are essential to a healthy life. They provide the energy our bodies and brains need to function properly. Carbs are primarily divided into two types:

1. Complex carbohydrates—starches and fiber found in fruits, vegetables, grains, and legumes.
2. Simple carbohydrates—sugars found in dairy products, white sugar, honey, fruit, maple syrup, raw sugar, and sweet vegetables.

Deficiencies in the enzymes needed to digest sugars and starches can be the result of eating too much of that type of food or an inherent enzyme insufficiency. In most cases, however, I believe that the main problem is eating too many carbs, particularly white pastas, breads, and sweets of all kinds. In the early 20th century, the average person consumed approximately 5 pounds of sugar per year; currently, the amount consumed is 150 pounds per year. Obviously, our bodies are not that different from our great-grandparents' and cannot handle a 30-fold increase in the amount of sugar we eat. Our bodies must attempt to keep up with the increased enzyme load but, over time, this burden takes its toll, resulting in an intolerance to sugars or carbohydrates or both, brought on largely because the enzymes we need to digest carbs have been depleted.

Different People, Different Diets

When I explain enzyme deficiencies and depletion to my clients or during media interviews, undoubtedly someone asks, "How much is the right amount of sugar to eat?" or "How much protein should I eat?" The reality is that there is no average amount that is suitable for all people. The old adage that "one person's food is another's poison" really holds true when it comes to food. One person may be able to tolerate sugar much better than another. While everyone needs protein, sugars (from healthy sources), fatty acids, vitamins, and minerals, we differ in how much of each we need.

Think about meat consumption. About 10 percent of our ancestors' diet was made up of animal protein, whereas we average 248 pounds of meat every year, or about 40 percent of our total caloric intake. When we take in more protein, our bodies need to increase protease production, a task that may not be possible. And doing so over time can lessen the amount of protease that is available for other important tasks in the body. Remember that protease also plays a role in our immune systems by killing pathogens and even cancer cells.

So you can easily see how your diet may be a significant part of the problem in depleting your enzymes. But you need to know which dietary issue you're most likely to experience so you can correct it. In some cases, it might already give you a clue as to your Phytozyme Cure Type. For example, you admit that you eat quite a lot of bread (that would be my husband, a real "bread head"). If that's the case, you're probably a Phytozyme Cure Carb Type. If meat is your downfall or you're eating a high protein diet, you're probably a Phytozyme Cure Protein Type. If you crave fatty foods, you're probably deficient in fatty acids, which makes you a Phytozyme Cure Fat Type.

Just remember, a Phytozyme Cure Fat Type is not necessarily someone who is overweight. You can be skinny and still be a Fat Type. This type does not reflect the shape or size of your body, but rather how well your body digests fats and fatty foods, and whether you may have a deficiency in lipase, the enzyme responsible for fat digestion.

The Phytozyme Cure Carb Type

The Phytozyme Cure Carb Type can be linked to a deficiency in one or more enzymes, including amylase (the primary type of enzyme that is involved with carb digestion), as well as sucrase, lactase, and maltase (the enzymes that digest sugar, milk sugar, and malt respectively). A deficiency in one or more of these enzymes can be caused from overconsumption of carbohydrate and sugary foods, an inherent deficiency of enzymes, or a combination of both.

Quiz: The Phytozyme Cure Carb Type

Are you deficient in enzymes such as amylase that digest complex carbohydrates or sugars (also known as simple carbohydrates)? I designed this quiz to help you find out. Here are some of the symptoms and health conditions that can be linked to a deficiency in one or more of these enzymes. Give yourself one point for each condition or symptom that you currently experience. If you experienced it as a child or even a year ago, do not give yourself a point. This is about right now. At the end of this section, make a note of your total points for this Phytozyme Cure Type, which you'll refer to momentarily.

- Abdominal cramps
- Abscesses (with pus)
- ADHD (attention-deficit/hyperactivity disorder) or ADD (attention deficit disorder)
- Aggression or violent behavior
- Allergies
- Allergies to bee stings or bug bites, poison ivy or oak
- Asthma
- Bipolar syndrome (manic depression)
- Bloating within two hours of eating a meal
- Body odor
- Bronchitis (recurring)
- Canker sores
- Celiac or gluten sensitivity/intolerance (confirmed by laboratory testing)
- Chicken pox
- Cold extremities
- Colic
- Cravings for breads, pastries, or sweets
- Depression
- Diarrhea, especially after eating dairy products
- Dizziness, especially when bending over
- Eczema (weeping)
- Environmental illness
- Excessive muscle soreness or pain after exercise
- Fatigue
- Flatulence (frequently)
- Herpes 1 or 2
- Hives
- Hypoglycemia
- Inflammation
- Insomnia
- Irritability or anger
- Mood swings

- Muscle and joint stiffness that is worse in the morning
- Neck and/or shoulder pain
- Nightmares (excessive)
- Panic attacks
- Premenstrual syndrome (PMS)
- Psoriasis
- Rashes
- Schizophrenia
- Seizure disorders
- Shingles
- Writer's cramps (cramps in your hands while writing)

The Phytozyme Cure Fat Type

Before you panic, thinking, "I hope I'm not a Fat Type!" remember that being this type has nothing to do with being overweight. Whether you're a Phytozyme Cure Fat Type depends on whether you may be lacking fat-digesting enzymes or eating more fatty foods than your body can handle, or both. However, a deficiency in fat-digesting enzymes, such as lipase, may be linked to excess weight or obesity, because an overweight body does not metabolize fats properly. But it is still possible to be a Phytozyme Cure Fat Type and be underweight or a healthy body weight.

Quiz: The Phytozyme Cure Fat Type

Are you deficient in fat-digesting enzymes, such as the enzyme lipase? I designed this quiz to help you find out. Here are some of the symptoms and health conditions that can be linked to a deficiency in this important enzyme. Give yourself one point for each condition or symptom that you currently experience. If you experienced it a year ago or as a child, do not give yourself a point. This is about right now. At the end of this section, make a note of your total points for this Phytozyme Cure Type, so you can refer to it later on.

- Achy feet
- Acne
- Arthritis
- Bladder problems
- Constipation
- Cystitis
- Diabetes type 1 or 2
- Diarrhea
- Difficulty losing weight
- Dizziness when altering bodily positions
- Excessive belching and/or nausea after eating
- Gallstones or had gallstone surgery
- Hay fever
- Heart disease
- Heart problems
- High blood pressure or taking antihypertension medications
- High cholesterol
- High triglycerides
- Intolerance of fatty or spicy foods
- Low stomach acid (hypochlorohydria)
- Ménière's disease
- Obesity
- Prostate problems
- Psoriasis
- Varicose veins
- Viruses (recurring)

The Phytozyme Cure Protein Type

If you eat a high-protein diet, as many people do, your body may become depleted in the enzymes, particularly protease, that digest these foods. Meats of all kinds require vast amounts of energy and enzymes to digest them, so you may be particularly prone to protease deficiency if you eat meat at most meals. While heavy meat eaters will more likely be Protein Types than vegetarians, you can still be a vegetarian Protein Type. Some people's bodies simply have insufficient protease, no matter what food groups they prefer. If you're like most people, you're probably worrying, "If I eat less meat, how will I get protein into my diet?" Trust me, there's no need to worry. Many fruits, vegetables, grains, nuts, and seeds are excellent sources of protein. However, while a Protein Type is well advised to cut back on meat, you don't have to become a vegetarian if that isn't right for you.

Quiz: The Phytozyme Cure Protein Type

Are you deficient in protein-digesting enzymes, such as important protease enzymes, which are linked to protein digestion? Simply take this quiz to find out. Here are some of the symptoms and health conditions that may be linked to a deficiency. Give yourself one point for each condition or symptom that you currently experience. If you experienced it a year ago or as a child, do not give yourself a point. This is about right now. At the end of this section, make a note of your total points for this Phytozyme Cure Type so you can refer to it later on.

- Acute pancreatitis
- AIDS
- Anxiety
- Appendicitis
- Arthritis
- Back weakness
- Bacterial or viral infections
- Blood clots

- Bone spurs
- Calcium deficiency
- Cancer
- Cold hands and feet
- Colon cancer
- Constipation
- Disc problems
- Edema (water retention) in hands or ankles
- Fluid in ears
- Fungal infections
- Gingivitis
- Gout
- Gum disorders
- Hearing loss
- Hypertension
- Hypoglycemia
- Insomnia
- Kidney disease or nephritis
- Mood swings
- Osteoporosis
- Parasitic infections
- Rashes
- Soft tissue damage (either traumatic or surgical)
- Tooth decay

Your Quiz Scores

Write down your total points for each Phytozyme Cure Type quiz here:

- Carb Type   _____
- Fat Type   _____
- Protein Type   _____

What Your Scores Mean

If one of your scores is much higher than the others, that probably indicates your Phytozyme Cure Type. For example, my client Judy's scores were Carb Type—10, Fat Type—2, and Protein Type—5. Because Judy had the most points in the Carb Type quiz, she is a Carb Type, and she would follow the dietary suggestions in the Phytozyme Cure Carb Type Diet later in this chapter. If you found you had the highest scores on the Fat Type quiz, then you're a Fat Type, and you should follow the dietary suggestions that apply to you. And if you find you're a Protein Type, see the Phytozyme Cure Protein Type Diet for dietary suggestions I've made just for you.

The Phytozyme Cure Combination Type

But what if your scores look more like those of my client Dan? Dan's scores were Carb Type—15; Fat Type—12; and Protein Type—13. There's no clear type, but aspects of all three types are present. That makes Dan a Combination Type. If your scores are close (within two or three points of each other), you are likely a Phytozyme Cure Combination Type too, and you can follow the Phytozyme Cure Combination Type Diet that I provide a bit later in this chapter.

And if you're not sure what type you are, don't worry! The Phytozyme Cure still applies to you. If you really don't know which dietary suggestions to follow, choose the Phytozyme Cure Combination Type. Stick to it for a couple of months and then take the quizzes again to see if there is a clear type pattern that presents itself at that time.

Regardless your type, be sure to keep track of your Phytozyme Type quiz scores, since you'll be using them to customize your Phytozyme Cure and to fine-tune your program further to suit a specific health condition in Part Two of this book. Or you may just want to refer back to them after a few months to see if anything has changed.

What Do Your Cravings Mean?

Talk about irony: the food that you are most likely to crave is also the one to which you may be intolerant or have difficulty digesting. It seems like our hardwiring is punishing us, but there's a reason why this happens. If you lack the enzymes to break down a particular type of food, your body may not get enough building blocks from that kind of food, causing you to crave more and more of it. For example, if you lack the enzyme lipase, your body won't get enough fatty acids, which are the building blocks of healthy fatty foods, so your body becomes deficient in fatty acids. In an effort to get more fatty acids into your diet, you keep experiencing cravings for fatty foods. But eating more fatty foods may not help. You may need to eat healthier fats and supplement with a digestive enzyme containing lipase to help your body break down the fatty foods into their fatty acid components. Think about these questions to find out what your cravings are telling you:

Do you crave sugar, bread, or pastries? You may have a sugar or carbohydrate intolerance or lack sufficient enzymes to digest them properly. You may need to cut back on unhealthy simple sugars. (Remember our discussion on simple carbs versus complex carbs?) By choosing beans or whole grains that keep your blood sugars stable for hours, you avoid the peaks and valleys that go hand in hand with eating sweets. And, by taking a digestive enzyme supplement containing some of the enzymes that break down carbs—including amylase, sucrase, lactase, and maltase— your body will obtain the fuel it needs.

Do you crave potato chips, corn chips, or cheese? You're probably intolerant of fats or have difficulty digesting them due to a lipase deficiency. Your body may also be deficient in essential fatty acids. Cut back on the unhealthy fatty foods—you know which ones they are. Choose small amounts of unsalted raw nuts, seeds, or avocado to include in your meals along with a digestive enzyme supplement containing lipase to help your body extract the essential fats found in these foods. Also, your body may crave fatty foods when you're experiencing chronic stress, so do your best to reduce your stress and implement some stress-management techniques into your day. They can include deep breathing, yoga, exercise, meditation, or just a nice long soak in the bathtub.

Do you crave steaks, eggs, chicken, or other types of meat? You may be intolerant of protein foods or have trouble breaking them down due to a protease deficiency. Most likely you experience some digestive upset immediately after eating protein foods or meat. Your body may lack the enzymes to extract the amino acids from protein foods, causing you to be deficient in these nutritional building blocks, no matter how much protein-rich food you eat. The best strategy is to eat protein foods in smaller amounts and supplement with a digestive enzyme containing protease with each meal to help your body break the protein down into amino acids.

Dietary Suggestions for Your Phytozyme Cure Type

In the next section you will learn about the specific foods to eat for your particular Phytozyme Cure Type. During the development of this plan, I discovered that Dr. Ellen Cutler had created an excellent dietary recommendation list in her book *Micro Miracles*. Combined with my research and modifications, it forms the dietary suggestions that follow. The food options listed under your type are tailored for your individual needs. By following the dietary suggestions listed for you, you'll give your body a much-needed break from foods that stress your body type. You'll also eat the foods that will help your body strengthen and rebuild, particularly if you have been experiencing any health challenges.

There are four diets described on the following pages; one for each Phytozyme Cure Type. Keep in mind that this is not about dieting; it's about following a healthy way of eating. While eating healthily for your type may take some effort, you will be rewarded with better health.

Many people want a food, herb, or drug that cures them. But remember our discussion about these Band-Aid approaches to health? They don't address the underlying problems causing the health concerns. By following the Type Diet recommended for you, you'll be addressing the root causes of your health concerns and giving your body the building blocks it needs. With this approach, it may take longer to experience symptom relief, but the relief will be long lasting.

The Phytozyme Cure Carbohydrate Type Diet[2]

By now you probably understand that there are two main reasons why someone is a Carb Type: either he or she consumes too many carbs like sweets, breads or pastas, or he or she has a weakness in manufacturing the enzymes required to digest carbs. It does not matter what the reason is, though, because the treatment is the same: a low-carb diet and supplementing with carbohydrate-digesting enzymes. That doesn't mean that you should start eating large amounts of meat, as some low-carb diets suggest. If you do, you may find yourself a Protein or Fat Type in the future.

Perhaps the two most common symptoms of being a Carb Type include bloating and gas within two hours of eating a meal and cravings for sugar or starch. People who are Carb Types may experience asthma, severe allergies, bloating, chronic constipation, depression, fatigue, and/or PMS. To help restore balance to the Carb Type, it is important to:

1. Limit consumption of alcohol.
2. Limit consumption of sugars or sugary foods, white breads, pastas, sweet vegetables like carrots and corn, dairy products, and fruit.

3. Eat plentiful amounts of vegetables.
4. Eat moderate amounts of healthy fats, and plant and animal proteins.
5. Avoid artificial sweeteners and food additives (all dietary types should do this).
6. Dramatically reduce your intake of caffeinated beverages and caffeine-containing foods like chocolate.
7. Avoid most grains. Whole grains are the exception, however, and they include wild rice, brown rice, buckwheat, kamut, spelt, and quinoa. You can still eat bread and pasta made from these grains. Be aware that most whole-grain bread is white bread with a handful of whole grains added and is not part of *The Phytozyme Cure* program. The label should state "100% whole grain" and not simply "whole grain."

So you've cleaned up your eating habits, you know your Phytozyme Cure Type, and you're ready to transform your health. Now, you'll start to incorporate the best foods for your type into your diet.

In the following table you'll see the number of servings for a particular type of food and the specific foods suitable for the Phytozyme Cure Carbohydrate Type. Unless specified otherwise, a serving of fruit is a single piece (in the case of an apple or pear, for example), or approximately 1/2 cup. For meat, poultry, and fish, a serving is about 4 ounces. For example, the Carb Type diet suggests three to five servings of protein foods a day and three to five servings of grains. While that may be more protein and fewer carbs than you're used to eating, it is important to focus on protein foods that help stabilize blood sugar levels while downplaying carbs, since most Carb Types eat excessive amounts of sugary foods, pastas, and breads. If you don't see a particular food listed in the table, that probably means you should avoid it.

Here are the dietary suggestions for the Carb Type:

Food Type	Foods and Number of Servings
Protein (1 serving = 4 ounces unless stated otherwise)	*3 to 5 servings/day unless stated otherwise* Beef (lean, 3 or fewer servings/week) Eggs (1) Fish Lamb Legumes Poultry Seeds Shellfish Soy or dairy yogurt Soy protein powder Spirulina or green protein Tofu
Vegetables in unlimited quantities	*Unlimited servings/day* Alfalfa sprouts Arugula Asparagus Bean sprouts Beans, green and yellow Bok choy Broccoflower Broccoli Brussels sprouts Cabbage Cauliflower Celery Collard greens Cucumbers Dandelion greens Endive Escarole Jicama Kale Kohlrabi Leeks Lettuce Mustard greens

Okra
Onions
Peppers, bell
Peppers, hot (fresh, not pickled)
Radishes
Rutabaga
Sea vegetables (such as agar, arame, dulse, hijiki, and nori)
Sorrel
Spinach
Sprouts (other types)
Squash
Tomatoes
Turnips
Watercress
Zucchini

Vegetables in limited quantities

3 to 4 servings/week

Carrots
Corn
Peas
Potatoes, white and red
Pumpkin
Sweet potatoes
Yams

Fats

2 servings/day

Almond butter (1/2 tsp)
Almonds (10)
Avocado (1/2 tbsp)
Olive oil (1/3 tsp)
Olive oil and vinegar dressing (1 tsp)
Olives (3)
Tahini (sesame butter) (1/2 tbsp)

Fats

3 to 4 servings/week

Brazil nuts (2)
Butter (1/3 tsp)
Mayonnaise (real, no chemicals)
Peanut butter (1/2 tbsp)
Sesame oil (1/2 tsp)
Walnuts (1/2 tsp)

Continued on page 126

Continued from page 125

Food Type	Foods and Number of Servings
Grain and legumes	*3 to 4 servings/day*
	Beans and lentils (all kinds, 1/3 cup cooked)
	Buckwheat (1/2 cup cooked)
	Corn tortilla (1)
	Popcorn (2 cups popped)
	Quinoa (1/2 cup cooked)
	Spelt (1/2 cup cooked)
	Wild rice (1/2 cup cooked)
Fruit	*2 servings/day*
	Apples
	Apricots
	Berries
	Cantaloupe
	Cherries
	Cranberries
	Grapefruit
	Grapes
	Honeydew melon
	Nectarines
	Peaches
	Pears
	Pineapple
	Plums
	Tangerines
	Watermelon

The Phytozyme Cure Fat Type Diet[2]

A person who needs a Fat Type Diet typically feels sluggish after eating meat and is prone to fluid retention, constipation, mood swings, or other symptoms linked to low blood sugar levels. He or she may also be deficient in fatty acids because the body is struggling to extract them from food or because he or she chooses to eat the wrong kinds of fats.

To help restore balance to the Fat Type, it is important to:

1. Limit consumption of alcohol.
2. Limit consumption of sugars or sugary foods, white breads, pastas, sweet vegetables like carrots and corn, dairy products, and fruit.
3. Eat plentiful amounts of vegetables.
4. Eat moderate amounts of healthy fats, and plant and animal proteins.
5. Avoid artificial sweeteners and food additives (all dietary types should do this).
6. Dramatically reduce your intake of caffeinated beverages and caffeine-containing foods like chocolate.
7. Avoid most grains. Whole grains are the exception, however, and they include wild rice, brown rice, buckwheat, kamut, spelt, and quinoa. You can still eat bread and pasta made from these grains. Be aware that most whole-grain bread is white bread with a handful of whole grains added and is not part of *The Phytozyme Cure* program. The label should state "100% whole grain" and not simply "whole grain."

Now that you've cleaned up your eating habits, are armed with your Phytozyme Cure Type, and are ready to transform your health, it's time to incorporate the best foods for your type into your diet. In the following table you'll see the number of servings for a particular type of food and the specific foods suitable for the Phytozyme Cure Fat Type. Unless specified otherwise, a serving of fruit is a single piece (in the case of an apple or pear, for example) or approximately 1/2 cup. For meat, poultry, and fish, a serving is about 4 ounces. For Fat Types, I suggest one to two servings of protein foods daily. That may actually be less meat than you're used to eating, but the emphasis for the Fat Type is on vegetables and fruits to reduce the amount of fatty foods you're ingesting. If you don't see a particular food on the table, that probably means you should avoid it.

Here are the dietary suggestions and food options for the Fat Type:

Food Type	Foods and Number of Servings
Protein (1 serving = 4 ounces unless stated otherwise)	*1 to 2 servings/day unless stated otherwise* Beef (lean) Chicken Eggs (3 or fewer/week) Fish Legumes Poultry Shellfish Soy or dairy yogurt Soy protein powder Soybeans Spirulina or green protein Tofu
Vegetables in unlimited quantities	*Unlimited servings/day* Alfalfa sprouts Arugula Asparagus Bean sprouts Beans, green and yellow Bok choy Broccoflower Broccoli Brussels sprouts Cabbage Cauliflower Celery Collard greens Cucumbers Dandelion greens Endive Escarole Jicama Kale Kohlrabi Leeks Lettuce

Mustard greens
Okra
Onions
Peppers, bell
Peppers, hot (fresh, not pickled)
Pumpkin
Radishes
Rutabaga
Sea vegetables (such as agar, arame,
dulse, hijiki, and nori)
Sorrel
Spinach
Sprouts (other types)
Tomatoes
Turnips
Watercress
Yellow squash
Zucchini

Vegetables in limited quantities	*3 to 4 servings/week*
	Carrots
	Corn
	Peas
	Potatoes, white and red
	Sweet potatoes
	Yams
Fats	*2 servings/day*
	Almond butter (1/2 tsp)
	Almonds (10)
	Avocado (1/2 tbsp)
	Olive oil (1/4 tsp)
	Olive oil and vinegar dressing (1 tsp)
	Olives (3)
	Tahini (sesame butter) (1/2 tbsp)
Fats	*3 to 4 servings/week*
	Brazil nuts (2)
	Butter (1/3 tsp)
	Mayonnaise (real, no chemicals)
	Peanut butter (1/2 tbsp)
	Sesame oil (1/2 tsp)
	Walnuts (1/2 tsp)

Continued on page 130

Continued from page 129

Food Type	Foods and Number of Servings
Grain and legumes	*2 servings/day*
	Beans and lentils (all kinds, 1/3 cup cooked)
	Buckwheat (1/2 cup cooked)
	Buckwheat noodles (1/2 cup cooked)
	Corn tortilla (1)
	Quinoa (1/2 cup cooked)
	Wild rice (1/3 cup cooked)
Fruit	*3 servings/day*
	Apples
	Apricots
	Berries
	Cantaloupe
	Cherries
	Cranberries
	Dates
	Figs
	Grapefruit
	Grapes
	Honeydew melon
	Nectarines
	Peaches
	Pears
	Pineapple
	Plums
	Tangerines
	Watermelon

The Phytozyme Cure Protein Type Diet[2]

The Protein Type tends to have difficulty digesting excessive amounts of protein foods or eats too many of them for his or her body to handle.

To help restore balance to the Protein Type, it is important to:

1. Limit consumption of alcohol.
2. Limit consumption of sugars or sugary foods, white breads, pastas, sweet vegetables like carrots and corn, dairy products, and fruit.

3. Eat plentiful amounts of vegetables.

4. Eat moderate amounts of healthy fats, and plant and animal proteins.

5. Avoid artificial sweeteners and food additives (all dietary types should do this).

6. Dramatically reduce your intake of caffeinated beverages and caffeine-containing foods like chocolate.

7. Avoid most grains. Whole grains are the exception, however, and they include wild rice, brown rice, buckwheat, kamut, spelt, and quinoa. You can still eat bread and pasta made from these grains. Be aware that most whole-grain bread is white bread with a handful of whole grains added and is not part of *The Phytozyme Cure* program. The label should state "100% whole grain" and not simply "whole grain."

So, you've cleaned up your eating habits, determined your Phytozyme Cure Type, and you're ready to transform your health. Now, you'll incorporate the best foods for your type into your diet. In the following table you'll see the number of servings for a particular type of food and the specific foods suitable for the Phytozyme Cure Protein Type. Unless specified otherwise, a serving of fruit is a single piece (in the case of an apple or pear, for example) or approximately 1/2 cup. For meat, poultry, and fish, a serving is about 4 ounces.

I suggest one to two servings of protein foods daily for the Protein Type. That may actually be less protein than you're used to. But the Protein Type tends to eat excessive amounts of protein foods for his or her body, thereby depleting the body's protease enzyme stores—so yes, you need to eat more vegetables. If you don't like them, now is the time to start trying them in different ways. (As I tell my clients, my husband couldn't stand most vegetables when we met, but after showing him how delicious they can be prepared with herbs and spices for added flavor, he now loves most kinds of veggies.) If you don't see a particular food listed on the table, that probably means you should avoid it.

Here are the dietary suggestions and food options for the Protein Type:

Food Type	Foods and Number of Servings
Protein (1 serving = 4 ounces unless stated otherwise)	*1 to 2 servings/day unless stated otherwise* Beef (lean) Chicken Eggs (3 or fewer/week) Fish Legumes Poultry Shellfish Soy or dairy yogurt Soy protein powder Soybeans Spirulina or green protein Tofu
Vegetables in unlimited quantities	*Unlimited servings/day* Alfalfa sprouts Arugula Asparagus Bean sprouts Beans, green and yellow Bok choy Broccoflower Broccoli Brussels sprouts Cabbage Cauliflower Celery Collard greens Cucumbers Dandelion greens Endive Escarole Jicama Kale Kohlrabi Leeks

	Lettuce
	Mustard greens
	Okra
	Onions
	Peppers, bell
	Peppers, hot (fresh, not pickled)
	Pumpkin
	Radishes
	Rutabaga
	Sea vegetables (such as agar, arame, dulse, hijiki, and nori)
	Sorrel
	Spinach
	Sprouts (other types)
	Tomatoes
	Turnips
	Watercress
	Yellow squash
	Zucchini
Vegetables in limited quantities	*3 to 4 servings/week*
	Carrots
	Corn
	Peas
	Potatoes, white and red
	Sweet potatoes
	Yams
Fats	*2 servings/day*
	Almond butter (1/2 tsp)
	Almonds (10)
	Avocado (1/2 tbsp)
	Olive oil (1/4 tsp)
	Olive oil and vinegar dressing (1 tsp)
	Olives (3)
	Tahini (sesame butter) (1/2 tbsp)
Fats	*3 to 4 servings/week*
	Brazil nuts (2)
	Butter (1/3 tsp)
	Mayonnaise (real, no chemicals)
	Peanut butter (1/2 tbsp)
	Sesame oil (1/2 tsp)
	Walnuts (1/2 tsp)

Continued on page 134

Continued from page 133

Food Type	Foods and Number of Servings
Grain and legumes	2 servings/day
	Beans and lentils (all kinds, 1/3 cup cooked)
	Buckwheat (1/2 cup cooked)
	Buckwheat noodles (1/2 cup cooked)
	Corn tortilla (1)
	Quinoa (1/2 cup cooked)
	Wild rice (1/3 cup cooked)
Fruit	3 servings/day
	Apples
	Apricots
	Berries
	Cantaloupe
	Cherries
	Cranberries
	Dates
	Figs
	Grapefruit
	Grapes
	Honeydew melon
	Nectarines
	Peaches
	Pears
	Pineapple
	Plums
	Tangerines
	Watermelon

The Phytozyme Cure Combination Type Diet[2]

The Phytozyme Cure Combination Type shows no clear enzyme dominance. The dietary suggestions are a blend of the suggestions for all three types. The key to health and healing for the Combination Type is moderation: moderate amounts of carbs, protein, and fats. Excesses of any food type will throw the Combination Type out of balance. After following the Phytozyme Cure Combination Type diet for several months, I encourage you to go back and take the quizzes again to see if you have experienced any changes. Sometimes a person's body is just so out of balance that they do not fall into one clear type, but that person's true type may emerge after experimenting with dietary changes for a few months.

To help restore balance to the Combination Type, it is important to:

1. Limit consumption of alcohol.
2. Limit consumption of sugars or sugary foods, white breads, pastas, sweet vegetables like carrots and corn, dairy products, and fruit.
3. Eat plentiful amounts of vegetables.
4. Eat moderate amounts of healthy fats, and plant and animal proteins.
5. Avoid artificial sweeteners and food additives (all dietary types should do this).
6. Dramatically reduce your intake of caffeinated beverages and caffeine-containing foods like chocolate.
7. Avoid most grains. Whole grains are the exception, however, and they include wild rice, brown rice, buckwheat, kamut, spelt, and quinoa. You can still eat bread and pasta made from these grains. Be aware that most whole-grain bread is white bread with a handful of whole grains added and is not part of *The Phytozyme Cure* program. The label should state "100% whole grain" and not simply "whole grain."

By now you've cleaned up your eating habits, determined that you're a Combination Type, and you're ready to transform your health. Start by incorporating the best foods for your type into your diet. I've specified which ones are best for the Combination Type and the recommended number of servings daily. Unless specified otherwise, a serving of fruit is a single piece (one apple or pear, for example) or approximately 1/2 cup. For meat, poultry, and fish, a serving is about 4 ounces. For Combination Types, I recommend two to three servings of protein foods a day. That's because, with the Combination Type, your diet is all about moderation. No single type of food, other than vegetables, is emphasized. Instead, you'll be eating a wide variety of wholesome foods to prevent depletion of any type of enzyme. If you don't see a particular food on the table, that probably means you should avoid it.

Following are the dietary suggestions and food options for the Combination Type:

Food Type	Foods and Number of Servings
Protein (1 serving = 4 ounces unless stated otherwise)	*2 to 3 servings/day unless stated otherwise*
	Beef (lean, 3 or fewer servings/week)
	Eggs (3 or fewer/week)
	Fish
	Legumes
	Poultry
	Seeds
	Shellfish
	Soy or dairy yogurt
	Soy protein powder
	Spirulina or green protein
	Tofu
Vegetables in unlimited quantities	*Unlimited servings/day*
	Alfalfa sprouts
	Arugula
	Asparagus
	Bean sprouts
	Beans, green and yellow
	Bok choy
	Broccoflower
	Broccoli
	Brussels sprouts
	Cabbage
	Cauliflower
	Celery
	Collard greens
	Cucumbers
	Dandelion greens
	Endive

Escarole
Jicama
Kale
Kohlrabi
Leeks
Lettuce
Mustard greens
Okra
Onions
Peppers, bell
Peppers, hot (fresh, not pickled)
Pumpkin
Radishes
Rutabaga
Sea vegetables (such as agar, arame, dulse, hijiki, and nori)
Sorrel
Spinach
Sprouts (other types)
Tomatoes
Turnips
Watercress
Yellow squash
Zucchini

Vegetables in limited quantities

3 to 4 servings/week

Carrots
Corn
Peas
Potatoes, white and red
Sweet potatoes
Yams

Fats

2 servings/day

Almond butter (1/2 tsp)
Almonds (10)
Avocado (1/2 tbsp)
Olive oil (1/4 tsp)
Olive oil and vinegar dressing (1 tsp)
Olives (3)
Tahini (sesame butter) (1/2 tbsp)

Continued on page 138

Continued from page 137

Food Type	Foods and Number of Servings
Fats	*3 to 4 servings/week*
	Brazil nuts (2)
	Butter (1/3 tsp)
	Mayonnaise (real, no chemicals)
	Peanut butter (1/2 tbsp)
	Sesame oil (1/2 tsp)
	Walnuts (1/2 tsp)
Grain and legumes	*2 servings/day*
	Beans and lentils (all kinds, 1/3 cup cooked)
	Buckwheat (1/2 cup cooked)
	Buckwheat noodles (1/2 cup cooked)
	Corn tortilla (1)
	Quinoa (1/2 cup cooked)
	Wild rice (1/3 cup cooked)
Fruit	*2 servings/day*
	Apples
	Apricots
	Berries
	Cantaloupe
	Cherries
	Cranberries
	Grapefruit
	Grapes
	Honeydew melon
	Nectarines
	Peaches
	Pears
	Pineapple
	Plums
	Tangerines
	Watermelon

As you've learned from discovering your Phytozyme Cure Type, this is not a one-size-fits-all approach to healing. You are a unique person with unique strengths and weaknesses, so why should you be following the same diet and lifestyle as everyone else? Now that you've learned how to customize your food choices and the amounts of specific foods for your body, it's time to customize your food and supplement choices even further.

In Part Two you'll learn about the best phytonutrients, enzymes, and natural medicines for your particular health conditions and concerns. You'll continue to stick with the Phytozyme Cure Type diet that you've just learned, but you'll also add supportive foods and enzymes to maximize the healing results you'll experience.

PART **TWO**

The Phytozyme Cure for Specific Health Conditions

Using Plant Nutrients to Heal and Prevent Illness

Everyone has a doctor in him or her; we just have to help it in its work. The natural healing force within each one of us is the greatest force in getting well.
—Hippocrates

By now you've learned about the healing power of phytonutrients and enzymes, determined your Phytozyme Cure Type, and made some important dietary adjustments so your body can get the most out of the nutrients you need to live. Congratulations on the progress you've made! You're probably feeling more energetic and have noticed some of your symptoms are improving.

The Phytozyme Cure does not present a one-size-fits-all approach to health—particularly when it comes to the nutrients we need to heal our specific health concerns. That's what Part Two is all about: using your newfound knowledge to target any health conditions you may have.

Just remember that if you have any of the symptoms described in *The Phytozyme Cure,* and you have not yet gotten a medical diagnosis from a trained physician, it's important that you do so immediately. You need an accurate medical diagnosis so you can explore all the potential treatments and cures that are available to you. And an accurate diagnosis will help you choose the best natural options for your condition, as well.

Varying Your Diet

Throughout Part Two, I recommend many phytonutrients, enzymes, and other natural medicines. Don't worry: I don't expect you to take all of them. As I said, everyone is different, which is why I have listed many different options. One person may benefit from a particular supplement, while someone else may be better served by another.

Regarding the phytonutrients, I encourage you to make a copy of the chart "Phytonutrients: What They Do and Where to Find Them" in Chapter 1 on page 32, highlight the most beneficial phytonutrients listed below for your specific health condition, put the chart on your fridge, and start adding the relevant food sources to your diet. Doing this is easier than you think. After a week it will probably have become second nature. Again, you don't have to eat every food listed; simply adding variety to your diet through the foods listed will help tremendously.

An important rule of thumb while adding the food sources of phytonutrients to your diet is that, whenever possible, you should always *choose the vegetable options,* and eat fruit *in moderation only.* While fruit is a health food, it tends to be high in sugars. Although these sugars are natural, they can still interfere with healing processes if you consume them in high quantities. Your Phytozyme Cure diet plan provides a daily recommended number of fruit servings. However, if you're having a strong sweet craving, always choose a piece of fruit over candy or anything with refined sugar.

Buying Enzyme Supplements

Do not be alarmed that I may have listed six or seven different types of enzyme supplements for your health condition. There are many excellent enzyme supplements on the market that blend two or more enzymes together. For example, one of my favorites is Wobenzym N. It is a combination of bromelain, chymotrypsin, pancreatin, papain, rutin, and trypsin. So, if you see any or all of these enzymes listed for your health condition, you could supplement with Wobenzym N. If you choose this enzyme formulation or another one that is enteric-coated, do not take other types of enzymes at the same time. For example, if you're taking Wobenzym N, do not take a full-spectrum digestive enzyme at the same time. Other enzymes can break down the enteric-coating, preventing the enzymes from reaching the intestinal tract in sufficient doses to have full therapeutic effect.

Alternatively, you can use a full-spectrum digestive enzyme that contains a variety of the enzymes listed for your particular condition. In addition to taking the supplement with meals, take them between meals on an empty stomach as well. Don't worry if there are additional enzymes in the supplement that are not listed under your health condition. There is no harm from taking enzymes that are not indicated for your condition. If your body can make use of them, it will. If it can't, they will simply pass through your bowels in your stools.

Keep in mind that it may take some time for you to notice symptom changes while using enzymes, phytonutrients, and other natural medicines. You may recall our discussion in Chapter 3 where I explained the importance of restoring balance in the body—not simply masking symptoms—for long-term health. Unlike drugs that address only symptoms, these natural remedies are going to the root cause to address underlying problems. You may not feel the effects immediately, but when you do start to reap the benefits of good nutrition and natural medicines, they will be long lasting.

As you learned in the earlier chapters, I recommend that everyone take a probiotic supplement on an empty stomach, usually before bed, and a digestive enzyme supplement with every meal and snack. In addition, I recommend that, regardless of your health condition, if finances permit, you take Cellfood Oxygen and nutrient supplement. Cellfood is a liquid nutritional supplement that contains 78 minerals, 34 enzymes, 17 amino acids, and oxygen in a readily absorbable form. I have used this supplement myself and recommended it to clients in my practice for many years with excellent results. Take 8 to 10 drops three times daily.

ADHD/ADD

Attention-deficit/hyperactivity disorder (ADHD), also referred to as attention deficit disorder (ADD), is defined as "age-inappropriate impulsiveness, lack of concentration, and sometimes, excess physical activity." [1] The disorder is associated with learning difficulties and a lack of social skills. Because there are no laboratory tests that accurately diagnose ADHD, it is controversial and often diagnosed incorrectly.

Symptoms of ADHD include mood swings, restlessness, impulsiveness, impaired memory, poor coordination, short attention span, inability to sit still, tantrums, difficulty completing age-appropriate tasks, learning disorders, difficulty concentrating, and/or speech disorders.

If a person experiences any or all of these symptoms, getting a medical diagnosis to rule out any other potentially serious afflictions is important. I am frequently astounded to hear parents talk about their ADHD child, only to learn that a physician has never diagnosed the child's condition. Equally shocking are the stories I hear about teachers who demand that children be put on medication for ADHD.

Many children and adults who have been diagnosed with ADHD may be suffering from food sensitivities and the neurotoxic reactions of food additives in processed, packaged, and prepared foods. Sugar intolerance, low thyroid function, excitotoxin-laden foods in the diet, environmental allergies, blood sugar fluctuations, nutritional deficiencies, heavy-metal toxicity, emotional stresses, and poor digestion or absorption can be implicated in ADHD.

But there is good news for the healing potential of natural medicine for this condition: I've observed the symptoms of ADHD disappear when a person returns to a natural-foods diet, the way Mother Nature intended us to eat.

The Phytozyme Cure for ADHD/ADD

The Diet

Most people suffering from ADHD/ADD are eating more carbohydrates and sugars than their body can handle or are suffering from a sugar intolerance. To address these issues, follow the Phytozyme Cure Carb Type diet outlined in Chapter 4. Proper nutrition is the most important treatment for ADHD and should emphasize vegetables and moderate amounts of fruit.

In addition to a low-sugar, low-carb diet, it is important to eliminate food additives, colors, and other artificial ingredients, which can trigger the symptoms of ADHD. And studies report that hyperactive children tend to have higher sugar consumption than other children.[2] In a study of 264 hyperactive children, more than three-quarters had abnormal sugar tolerance.[3] Some of the most common food sensitivities in ADHD sufferers are wheat, gluten, dairy, corn, chocolate, peanuts, citrus, soy, and most food colors and additives.

Even a small amount of these substances can significantly lessen the likelihood of symptom improvement. Some parents wrongly assume that *reducing* the amount of problem foods and additives their child's diet will improve symptoms. However, my experience indicates otherwise. To people suffering from ADHD, synthetic colors, preservatives, and flavor enhancers are like poison. Eating a whole-foods diet, devoid of artificial ingredients, is essential to the proper handling of this disorder, and needs to be maintained for at least a few months to see a noticeable improvement. This diet also needs to be continued to maintain improvements.

If you suffer from ADHD/ADD, add foods rich in the following phytonutrients to your diet: astaxanthin, curcumin, hesperetin, lycopene, naringin, pectin, proanthocyanidin, resveratrol, and tangeretin. See the chart "Phytonutrients: What They Do and Where to Find Them" on page 32 for more about these specific phytonutrients.

Supplementing the Diet

Frequently, people suffering from ADHD/ADD are deficient in the enzymes known as disaccharidases, namely sucrose, lactose, and maltose, that digest cane sugar, milk sugar, and grain sugar respectively. Supplementing with a high-quality digestive enzyme formula that includes these enzymes is beneficial in reversing the sugar intolerance found in ADHD/ADD. Take 1 to 3 enzyme capsules or tablets with every meal to help digest the naturally present sugars, even if you think the meal is devoid of them. (You find sugar in many foods that you wouldn't expect. See Chapter 3 for more about cutting it out of your diet.)

It can also be helpful to supplement with one or more of the following enzymes between meals on an empty stomach: lipase, papain, and superoxide dismutase (SOD). Start with 1 capsule or tablet of your chosen enzyme(s) on an empty stomach 20 minutes before or at least 1 hour after meals, three times daily. You can gradually increase that amount to 3 capsules or tablets at a time, three times daily, or more with the guidance of a nutritional medicine practitioner who is experienced in systemic enzyme therapy.

Add a multivitamin and mineral supplement that is devoid of the allergenic substances I noted in Chapter 3. Your body requires adequate amounts of disaccharidase enzymes, including niacin, vitamin B6, vitamin C, biotin, magnesium, and zinc, all of which can be found in a good-quality multiple supplement. Zinc is particularly deficient in those suffering from learning difficulties.[4]

In addition, here are some of the most common nutritional deficiencies found in ADHD sufferers. Let me explain what the supplements do and why they may be helpful:

- *Essential fatty acids like DHA and GLA:* These are necessary for healthy brain functioning. Take 500 to 1000 milligrams of DHA and 100 milligrams of GLA daily. These essential fats are found in black currant oil, borage oil, fish oil, and evening primrose oil.

- *B-complex vitamins:* This spectrum of vitamins is required for a healthy nervous system and brain. They help you relax and calm your nerves (particularly B6), without any sedative effects. Vitamin B6 is especially helpful for children suffering from ADHD, but it should be combined with an additional B-complex vitamin, since they work synergistically. Also, too high a dose of one B vitamin can deplete levels of the others. Adults or children five years and older can take 50 to 100 milligrams per day of a B-complex supplement (such supplements usually contain 50 to 100 milligrams of each of the B vitamins, with the exception of folate and vitamin B12, which are measured in micrograms, not milligrams).
- *Calcium and magnesium:* These important minerals are required for a healthy nervous system. They do their best work when taken together. Many people take calcium without taking magnesium, which can throw off a healthy balance in the nervous system. The dose depends on many factors, but typically 500 milligrams of calcium and 250 milligrams of magnesium twice daily is beneficial to relax the nervous system.
- *Phosphatidylserine (PS):* This is a naturally occurring substance needed in high concentrations in brain cells. Supplementing with 300 to 500 milligrams daily for a few months may be helpful prior to tapering off to a maintenance dose of 100 to 300 milligrams per day. A study of 21 young people, aged 4 to 19, with ADHD found that supplementing with the nutrient phosphatidylserine (PS) helped over 90 percent of cases, especially improving attention and learning capacity. The dose used in the study was between 200 and 300 milligrams.[5]

People suffering from ADHD often have an overgrowth of harmful bacteria and fungi in their intestines. So make sure you are supplementing with a probiotic, as outlined in Chapter 3, preferably containing *Lactobacillus acidophilus, Lactobacillus bulgaricus, Lactobacillus plantarum, Bifidobacteria,* and *Bifidobacteria bifidum.*

Allergies

No one knows for sure why an everyday substance is harmless to one person and has such strong effects on another. When a person with allergies inhales or ingests his or her particular allergens, such as tree pollens, animal dander, dust mites, or a particular food, the body signals the immune system to destroy the offender. In doing so, cells release histamine and other chemicals, causing the classic itchy eyes, scratchy throat, runny nose, and sinus congestion or headache, among other symptoms.

While the medical approach is to take antihistamines, most have side effects, such as drowsiness, or can aggravate heart arrhythmias. Not to mention that they are only treating the symptoms, not getting to the cause of the allergies. This is one area where *The Phytozyme Cure* really shines!

The Phytozyme Cure for Allergies
The Diet
Most people suffering from allergies are eating more carbohydrates and sugars than their bodies can handle or have a sugar intolerance. To address these issues, follow the Phytozyme Cure Carb Type diet outlined in Chapter 4.

However, allergies can be linked to a deficiency of the enzymes you need to digest any food type or due to eating too much of particular food type. So if the quizzes in Chapter 4 indicate that you are a Phytozyme Cure Fat or Protein Type, follow the diet for that particular type instead. If you couldn't determine a clear type, follow the Phytozyme Cure Combination Type diet.

Regardless of the type of allergy, regular exposure to allergens in the environment or in undigested food can weaken the body, making it vulnerable to other health conditions. Undigested food can leak into the bloodstream through the walls of the intestines and, once there, cause the immune system to overreact, as it views the food particle as an invader.

Frequently people with allergies have multiple enzyme deficiencies, typically from consuming too much of a particular type of food and from stresses on the enzyme mechanisms in the body. During the first two months of your diet, completely avoid all dairy products. Avoid sugars and sugary foods during this time too. Later on, you may be able to eat these foods occasionally, but avoid them for two months to give your body a break.

Emphasize foods that contain anthocyanin, curcumin, hesperetin, and quercetin in your diet. See the chart "Phytonutrients: What They Do and Where to Find Them" on page 32 for more about these specific phytonutrients.

As I've seen in my practice, simply following these dietary suggestions is often sufficient for most people to see a tremendous improvement in or complete elimination of their allergies.

Supplementing the Diet

Supplementing your diet with a high-quality full-spectrum digestive enzyme formula that includes amylase, lipase, and protease, among other enzymes, is beneficial. Take 1 to 3 enzyme capsules or tablets with every meal to help your body break down the carbohydrates, fats, and proteins in your food into the natural sugars, essential fatty acids, and amino acids needed for optimal healing.

It can also be helpful to supplement with one or more of the following enzymes between meals on an empty stomach: amylase, bromelain, chymotrypsin, mucolase, papain, protease, serrapeptidase, or superoxide dismutase (SOD), or a single product that includes some or all of these enzymes. Start with 1 capsule or tablet of your chosen enzyme(s) on an empty stomach 20 minutes before or at least 1 hour after meals, three times daily. You can gradually increase that amount to 3 capsules or tablets at a time, three times daily, or more with the guidance of a nutritional medicine practitioner experienced in systemic enzyme therapy.

For quick relief of allergy symptoms, take 2000 milligrams of vitamin C, three times daily, with at least 2 to 3 hours between doses. If you experience loose stools, reduce the dose slightly.

Supplementing with the phytonutrient quercetin is also frequently helpful since, like vitamin C, it has antihistamine effects. Usually quercetin supplements contain the enzyme bromelain, creating a powerful blend of allergy-reducing compounds. Take 400 milligrams of quercetin twice daily.

Alzheimer's Disease

Alzheimer's disease is a progressive brain disorder that starts with memory loss and eventually leads to full-blown dementia and death. There are many symptoms associated with this disease, including memory problems, confusion and disorientation, inability to manage basic tasks, hallucinations and delusions, episodes of violence and rage, episodes of childlike behavior, paranoia, depression, and mood swings.

Alzheimer's affects a part of the brain called the hippocampus, the location of memory and intellect. Neurons in the hippocampus become entangled, resulting in abnormal protein fragment formations (called plaques or amyloid plaques) and lost brain cells. Scientists are still unsure whether the tangles and plaque formations cause Alzheimer's disease or whether they are a side effect. They are also unsure why some people get Alzheimer's and others do not. In addition, wherever the plaques are formed in the brain, there is accompanying inflammation, making scientists question the role of inflammation in Alzheimer's.

The Phytozyme Cure for Alzheimer's Disease
The Diet
People suffering from Alzheimer's disease can be experiencing a deficiency in any or all of the enzymes needed to digest carbohydrates, fats, or proteins. If, after taking the quizzes in Chapter 4, you found that you were a Phytozyme Cure Carb, Fat, or Protein Type, follow the diet for that particular type. If there was no clear type, follow the Phytozyme Cure Combination Type diet.

Since free radical formation plays a role in Alzheimer's disease, it needs to be addressed in its treatment, and diet is one way to do this. Environmental toxins and metal exposures also appear to be implicated in brain diseases. (For more information on metal exposures and their elimination, consult my book *The Brain Wash*.) Studies at the University of Calgary have demonstrated that mercury vapors cause a degeneration of brain neurons and also cause lesions similar to those found in people with Alzheimer's disease. In addition, elevated levels of homocysteine, a by-product of protein digestion and metabolism, are implicated in Alzheimer's. (You can read more about homocysteine under the condition "Heart Disease" on page 207) Excessively high levels have been linked to diseases or problems we frequently associate with aging, including heart disease, wrinkling, and Alzheimer's. Enzymes and phytonutrients are excellent to address high levels of homocysteine.

Add foods rich in curcumin and resveratrol to your diet to help address inflammation. See the chart "Phytonutrients: What They Do and Where to Find Them" on page 32 for more about these specific phytonutrients.

Supplementing the Diet

Supplementing your diet with a high-quality full-spectrum digestive enzyme formula that includes amylase, lipase, and protease, among other enzymes, is beneficial. Take 1 to 3 enzyme capsules or tablets with every meal to help your body break down the carbohydrates, fats, and proteins in your food into the natural sugars, essential fatty acids, and amino acids needed for optimal healing. It can also be helpful to supplement with one or more of the following enzymes between meals on an empty stomach: bromelain, papain, protease, superoxide dismutase (SOD), or trypsin, or a single product that includes some or all of these enzymes. Start with 1 capsule or tablet of your chosen enzyme(s) on an empty stomach 20 minutes before or at least 1 hour after meals, three times daily. You can gradually increase that amount to 3 capsules or tablets at a time, three times daily, or more with the guidance of a nutritional medicine practitioner experienced in systemic enzyme therapy.

Specific nutrient deficiencies, including that of vitamin B1, B12, and folate, have also been linked with the progression of Alzheimer's disease. You can address these deficiencies with a multivitamin and mineral supplement and an additional 100-milligram B-complex supplement, taken with breakfast or lunch.

Arteriosclerosis

Arteriosclerosis is the hardening and thickening of the walls of arteries in the body. Fatty deposits and calcium buildup can be the culprits, as can high blood pressure, which causes the muscular walls of the arteries to thicken over time. And, as you may have guessed, thicker arteries can interfere with the proper movement of blood in your body. To address this condition through The Phytozyme Cure, follow the dietary, supplement, and lifestyle suggestions under "Heart Disease" on page 209.

Arthritis

Arthritis is a painful condition of the joints. There are many types of arthritis, including rheumatoid arthritis, which is inflammatory, and osteoarthritis, which is degenerative.

Rheumatoid arthritis primarily affects the tissue connecting bones to joints. It most commonly affects the hands but usually occurs in many places at once. It can even affect the whole body, including elbows, wrists, and knees. While rheumatoid arthritis usually starts in middle age, many younger people experience rheumatoid arthritis too. Although it is not commonly known, bacterial, protozoa, yeast, and fungal infections can be a factor in some cases of rheumatoid arthritis.

Osteoarthritis, also known as degenerative joint disease, occurs when the cartilage in the joints begins to deteriorate and wear away.

This deterioration can occur because of excess weight or joint injuries and can have a genetic component.

Two other common forms of arthritis are gout and ankylosing spondylitis (a type of spinal arthritis). Regardless of the type of arthritis you're experiencing, you can feel improvements by following *The Phytozyme Cure.*

The Phytozyme Cure for Arthritis
The Diet
Most people suffering from arthritis are eating more protein-rich foods or fatty foods than their body can handle. They may have inherent enzyme deficiencies preventing them from digesting these foods. To address these concerns, follow The Phytozyme Cure Fat Type or The Phytozyme Cure Protein Type diet outlined in Chapter 4. These diets recommend cutting back on meat and eating a predominantly vegetarian diet.

Many arthritics are suffering from food sensitivities that aggravate their condition. Some of the main food sensitivities that arthritics experience are corn, wheat, gluten, rye bread, pork (including bacon), beef, eggs, coffee, dairy products, chocolate, and oranges. I highly recommend eliminating these foods, as well as alcohol and fried foods, from your diet.

Emphasize foods that contain anthocyanins, astaxanthin, capsaicin, catechins, curcumin, hesperetin, resveratrol, and tannins in your diet. See the chart "Phytonutrients: What They Do and Where to Find Them" on page 32 for more about these specific phytonutrients. Of course, if a common allergen like oranges is listed as a food source for a particular phytonutrient, avoid that food.

In my experience, many arthritics are prone to severe pH imbalances, which I talk about in Chapter 2. They almost always test acidic. Adopting an alkalizing diet made up of about 70 percent vegetables and limited meat and dairy products can substantially help to reduce pain and other symptoms. The topic of pH balancing is quite comprehensive and requires a full book to do it justice. If you want to read more about pH balancing, consult my book *The Ultimate pH Solution*.

Supplementing the Diet

The power of enzymes really shines when it comes to dealing with arthritis. A study published in *Zeitschrift für Rheumatologie* reported that 62 percent of arthritic patients showed improvement with enzyme therapy.[6]

Supplementing your diet with a high-quality full-spectrum digestive enzyme formula that includes amylase, lipase, and protease, among other enzymes, is also beneficial. Take 1 to 3 enzyme capsules or tablets with every meal to help your body break down the carbohydrates, fats, and proteins in your food into the natural sugars, essential fatty acids, and amino acids needed for optimal healing.

It can also be helpful to supplement with one or more of the following enzymes between meals on an empty stomach: bromelain, chymotrypsin, papain, protease, serrapeptidase, superoxide dismutase (SOD), or trypsin, or a single product that includes some or all of these enzymes. Much research shows the enzyme blend Wobenzym N is beneficial for arthritis. Start with 3 to 5 capsules or tablets of your chosen enzyme(s) on an empty stomach 20 minutes before or at least 1 hour after meals, three times daily. You can gradually increase that amount under the guidance of a nutritional medicine practitioner experienced in systemic enzyme therapy.

Alternatively, take 1500 milligrams a day of bromelain in divided doses between meals to reduce inflammation. Taking 1000 milligrams of quercetin a day with meals can also reduce inflammation.

Many other supplements are helpful in easing arthritis:

- Vitamin D, 2000 IU (international units) daily.
- DHA-EPA from flaxseed oil or fish oil, 1000 to 3000 milligrams of fish or flax oil daily. That's about 500 milligrams of EPA and 360 milligrams of DHA daily if you choose an EPA-DHA–type product.

- Methylsulfonylmethane (MSM) occurs naturally in the body and is found in some foods, particularly green vegetables. Take 5000 milligrams daily to counter pain and inflammation. Because it has blood-thinning properties, avoid using MSM if you are taking pharmaceutical blood thinners.
- Niacinamide, 3000 milligrams daily. (Alternatively, you can use niacin, but divide the doses, as it can cause flushing.)
- Glucosamine sulfate can be helpful in alleviating pain after using it for two to three months. Take 500 milligrams three times daily.
- S-adenosylmethionine (SAMe) to help to protect the fluid surrounding the joints. Follow package directions for dosage information since there are many product variations.
- Coenzyme Q10 (CoQ10), 300 milligrams daily.
- Vitamin E, 800 IU daily.
- Devil's claw, an excellent anti-inflammatory and anti-pain herb; take it in capsules or as an extract, following dosage instructions for the brand you choose.
- Aloe vera juice, 2 ounces daily on an empty stomach in the morning.

Asthma

Asthma is a serious respiratory condition that interferes with a person's ability to breathe. An asthma attack can cause someone to suffocate unless they get emergency medical intervention. Some of the symptoms of asthma are wheezing, coughing, chest tightness, increased heart rate, sleep loss due to coughing and difficulty breathing, increased mucus flow, inflammation of the mucus linings of the lungs, and airway constriction in the bronchial muscles.

Typically, asthmatics have some combination of bronchial muscle spasms, excess mucus production, and mucus lining swelling. Symptoms are the results of allergies, environmental irritants, infection, cold air, hormonal imbalances, exertion, and stress.

A troubling fact is that the incidence of asthma is on the rise. By some accounts it has increased by over 33 percent in just one decade. Research suggests this is because of pollution, food additives, and people eating diets that are higher in meat and fat, which cause inflammation.

The Phytozyme Cure for Asthma
The Diet

Most people suffering from asthma are eating more carbohydrates and sugars than their body can handle, or they have a sugar intolerance. To address these concerns, follow the Phytozyme Cure Carb Type diet outlined in Chapter 4. Asthmatic children in particular may be intolerant to sugar in its many forms, such as cane sugar, lactose (milk sugar), maltose (grain sugar), corn syrup, honey, and fructose. Consuming moderate amounts of organic fruit, which contains natural sugars, is probably okay. Asthmatics should never eat artificial sweeteners (aspartame, saccharin, and mannitol) or sorbitol.

Emphasize foods that contain anthocyanins, catechins, curcumin, hesperetin, lycopene, quercetin, and resveratrol in your diet. See the chart "Phytonutrients: What They Do and Where to Find Them" on page 32 for more about these specific phytonutrients.

Many foods tend to cause mucus, so eliminating them from your diet is important. All dairy products, sugar, junk food, fried foods, and food additives can cause excess mucus formation in the lungs, chest tightness, and lung spasms. The most critical food additives to avoid include preservatives, tartrazine and other food colors (such as yellow dye number 5), sulfites, benzoates, nitrates and nitrites (usually found in smoked foods and luncheon meats), and monosodium glutamate (MSG).

MSG, the sneaky hidden food additive that I discussed in Chapter 3, goes by many names, so watch for it carefully when you're choosing what to eat. Although I do not recommend eating prepared foods, if you do buy them, steer clear of those with any of the following ingredients on the label: autolyzed yeast, calcium caseinate, gelatin, glutamate, glutamic acid, hydrolyzed protein, hydrolyzed soy protein, isolated soy protein, monopotassium glutamate, sodium caseinate, yeast extract, yeast food, or yeast nutrient.

Drinking at least 8 to 12 glasses of water, herbal teas, and soup broth per day helps dilute excess mucus so your body can get rid of it.

A Sigh of Relief

It is important for asthmatics to avoid being exposed to substances that might trigger their symptoms. If you suffer from this condition, stay away from dust and dust mites, animal dander, cigarette smoke, pollens, mold spores, fireplace smoke, and chemicals that off-gas from furniture, household products, fragrances and scented products, and office products. Also, avoid perfumes and fragrances in personal care, makeup, and hair care products.

And it might sound obvious, but if you smoke, either tobacco or marijuana, you must quit immediately if you wish to overcome the breathing problems linked to asthma. Equally important, avoid second-hand smoke as much as possible.

Supplementing the Diet

Supplement with a high-quality full-spectrum digestive enzyme, taking 1 to 3 capsules or tablets with each meal. Just be sure the product contains protease, amylase, lipase, and disaccharidases like sucrose, maltose, and lactose.

It can also be helpful to supplement with one or more of the following enzymes between meals on an empty stomach: bromelain, chymotrypsin, mucolase, papain, protease, superoxide dismutase (SOD), or trypsin, or a single product that includes some or all of these enzymes. Start with 1 capsule or tablet of your chosen enzyme(s) on an empty stomach 20 minutes before or at least 1 hour after meals, three times daily. You can gradually increase that amount to 3 capsules or tablets at a time, three times daily, or more with the guidance of a nutritional medicine practitioner who is experienced in systemic enzyme therapy. You can also take 100 milligrams of the coenzyme Q10 (also called CoQ10) daily.

To address a possible essential fatty acid deficiency, take 1 to 2 tablespoons of flaxseed oil or 4 to 8 grams of fish oil daily. The latter often goes by the name DHA-EPA or EPA-DHA.

Supplementing with additional antioxidant phytonutrients like beta-carotene, capsaicin, and epigallocatechin gallate (EGCG) can also be helpful. The latter is found in green tea. You may wish to drink 3 cups of green tea daily instead of taking EGCG supplements. Supplementing with 1000 milligrams of the phytonutrient quercetin daily can help with asthma due to its anti-inflammatory and anti-allergic effects.

Most asthmatics are also deficient in the minerals calcium and magnesium. Take 1000 milligrams of calcium and magnesium daily with meals or before bed. Or you can also take 250 milligrams of calcium and magnesium three to four times per day. Cut back if you start to experience excessively loose stools.

High doses of vitamin C can dramatically improve breathing. Vitamin C is a potent antihistamine and anti-inflammation nutrient that tends to be depleted during stress, including asthma attacks. Take 1000 to 2000 milligrams four times daily with at least 2 to 3 hours between doses, for a total dosage of up to 8000 milligrams daily. I usually recommend vitamin C in its alkaline form—as calcium ascorbate rather than the more common ascorbic acid. Reduce the dosage if you start to experience excessively loose stools.

Take 400 IU of a natural source vitamin E supplement, preferably taken as mixed tocopherols. This powerful antioxidant helps protect the lungs against toxins and their resulting damages.

N-acetyl cysteine (sometimes called NAC) helps to liquefy mucus in the bronchial tubes and is a potent antioxidant against free radical damage in the lungs. Take 500 to 600 milligrams two times daily.

There are many excellent herbal medicines to treat asthma. Try one for a few weeks. If you're not getting any results, try a different one:

- *Coltsfoot* clears out excess mucus from the lungs and bronchial tubes. It also soothes coughs, and protects and soothes mucus membranes. You can use 1 to 2 teaspoons of dried herb per 1 cup water for a tea, drunk three times daily, or use 1/2 to 1 teaspoon of tincture (the herb in an alcohol base, found in most health food stores), three times daily.

- *Elecampane* kills harmful bacteria while reducing coughs and expelling mucus in the respiratory tract. It can also help eliminate toxins from the lungs. Take 1 teaspoon of the herb per 1 cup of water in a tea (also called an infusion), three times daily, or take 1 to 2 milliliters of the tincture three times daily.

- *Ephedra* is a plant that is an excellent bronchodilator and which has been used for thousands of years. However, its natural form is unavailable from health food stores in Canada. The synthetic form, ephedrine, has many side effects, and it's best to avoid it. In some people ephedra can cause heart palpitations, so avoid it if you are prone to them. And because it has a stimulating effect, don't take ephedra in the evening.

- *Horehound* relaxes the muscles of the lungs while encouraging them to clear excess mucus. Taken as a tea or tincture (not in candy form) can be helpful with asthma. Take 1 teaspoon of dried herb per 1 cup of water in a tea, three times daily. Alternatively take 1/4 to 1/2 teaspoon of tincture three times daily.

- *Licorice root* is a natural anti-inflammatory herb that has antiviral effects and helps support the body's stress glands, the adrenals, which are often depleted in asthmatics. It can be taken in tea or tincture form. Add 1 teaspoon of the dried root to 3 cups of water, bring to a boil, and simmer over low heat, covered, for 15 minutes. (You can also buy convenient licorice tea bags, but be sure to buy tea bags that contain only licorice root, with no other ingredients to dilute the medicinal effects.) Drink 1 cup three times daily. Alternatively, take 1 teaspoon of the tincture two to three times daily.

- *Lungwort* clears catarrh from the upper respiratory tract and bronchial tubes, while helping to soothe the mucous membranes and lessen coughs. It combines well with coltsfoot and horehound. As a tea, mix 1 to 2 teaspoons of dried herb per 1 cup of water. Drink 1 cup three times daily. Alternatively, take 1/4 to 1 teaspoon of tincture three times a day.

- *Marshmallow* is soothing to the mucus membranes of the lungs. It can be taken as a tea or tincture. For a tea, infuse 1 teaspoon of dried herb in 1 cup of water. Drink 1 cup three times daily.

- *Mullein leaves and flowers* soothe mucus membranes in the respiratory tract while helping the body to expel excess mucus. It also reduces inflammation in the bronchial tubes and is helpful for coughs. Use 1 to 2 teaspoons of dried herb per 1 cup of water in a tea. Drink 1 cup three times daily. Or take 1/4 to 1 teaspoon of tincture three times a day.

- *Pleurisy root* is good for clearing out excess mucus from the lungs. It also has antispasmodic properties. For those suffering from a large amount of mucus or catarrh buildup, pleurisy root works best when combined with coltsfoot. Combine 1/2 to 1 teaspoon of dried herb per 1 cup of water for a tea. Drink 1 cup three times daily. Or take 1/4 to 1/2 teaspoon of tincture three times a day.

Bladder Infections

Also known as cystitis or urinary tract infections, bladder infections occur when the bladder becomes vulnerable to bacterial invasion. When the bladder is infected, the interior walls of this organ become inflamed, which causes the urgent and frequent need to urinate, even if there is little urine excreted. Sometimes there is pain or burning with urination, and low back or abdominal pain, nausea and vomiting, or fevers. Commonly treated with antibiotics, these drugs leave the bladder more vulnerable to future bacterial infections.

Women are far more likely than men to experience bladder infections, primarily due to anatomical differences. In women, it is fairly easy for intestinal or vaginal bacteria to enter the urethra—the tube that conducts urine out of the bladder—and up into the bladder.

Many factors can lead to bladder infections, including the frequent use of antibiotics, stress, pregnancy, sexual intercourse, use of contraceptive diaphragms, structural variations in people, hormonal imbalances, injuries, harmful intestinal bacteria like E. coli, vaginal infections, and poor diet.

The Phytozyme Cure for Bladder Infections

The Diet

Most people suffering from recurring bladder infections are usually eating more sugars or fats than their body can handle. To address these concerns, follow the Phytozyme Cure Carb Type diet or the Phytozyme Cure Fat Type diet, depending on your quiz results from Chapter 4.

Regardless of the diet you will be following, remember that sugar feeds microbes like bacteria and viruses. So avoid sugar as much as possible while you have a bladder or urinary tract infection.

Fresh cranberries and unsweetened cranberry juice have potent antibiotic and antiviral substances to help eliminate bacteria and viruses from the body. Avoid cranberry cocktails—they are loaded with sugar that actually feeds infectious organisms. Drink pure cranberry juice diluted 1:4 cranberry juice to water (one part cranberry juice to four parts water). If this drink is too tart, dilute it to a ratio of 1:1:3 cranberry juice to pure apple juice to water (one part cranberry juice, one part apple juice, three parts water). Choose a brand of juice without additives and preservatives. Alternatively, you can take 500 milligrams of cranberry extract capsules two times daily.

Emphasize foods that contain alpha-carotene, anthocyanins, beta-carotene, catechins, curcumin, hesperetin, tannins, and terpene limonoids in your diet. See the chart "Phytonutrients: What They Do and Where to Find Them" on page 32 for more about these specific phytonutrients to boost the immune system, reduce inflammation, and fight microbes.

Also, be sure you're drinking lots of pure water to help flush bacteria and toxins from the urinary tract.

Supplementing the Diet

Supplementing your diet with a high-quality full-spectrum digestive enzyme formula that includes amylase, lipase, and protease, among other enzymes, is also beneficial. Take 1 to 3 enzyme capsules or tablets with every meal to help your body break down the carbohydrates, fats, and proteins in your food into the natural sugars, essential fatty acids, and amino acids needed for optimal healing.

It can also be helpful to supplement with one or more of the following enzymes between meals on an empty stomach: bromelain, chymotrypsin, papain, protease, serrapeptidase, superoxide dismutase (SOD), or trypsin, or a single product that includes some or all of these enzymes. Start with 1 capsule or tablet of your chosen enzyme(s) on an empty stomach 20 minutes before or at least 1 hour after meals, three times daily. You can gradually increase that amount to 3 capsules or tablets at a time, three times daily, or more with the guidance of a nutritional medicine practitioner experienced in systemic enzyme therapy.

Although many people take vitamin C to avoid a deficiency, it is perhaps the most overlooked natural remedy for therapeutic purposes. Not only does it enhance immune system function, it inhibits the growth of E. coli and other bacteria so they cannot grow as readily. To help prevent bacteria-caused bladder infections, take 1000 milligrams five times a day in divided doses.

There are many excellent herbal medicines for bladder and urinary tract infections, but two of my favorites are aloe vera juice and oregano oil. Let's look at these remedies in more detail:

Aloe vera: This natural substance has been used safely for over four thousand years to heal bladder and urinary tract infections. It is antibacterial, antiviral, analgesic (pain-killing), anti-inflammatory, fever-reducing, and cleansing to the body, making it an excellent choice. Full of amino acids, enzymes, phytonutrients, essential oils, vitamins, and minerals, aloe vera helps nourish the body and its immune system while it directly deals with infection. Drink 1/4 cup of aloe vera juice twice a day. Note that aloe vera juice is not the same as aloe gel, which tends to be thicker and more concentrated. Avoid using "aloes" or "aloe latex," since these alternatives have purgative actions on the intestinal tract. Pregnant or lactating women should avoid drinking aloe vera juice.

Oregano oil: Research shows that this is one of the most potent antibacterial and antiviral substances you can take. In a study reported by *ScienceDaily* magazine, oil of oregano was found to be effective against staphylococcus bacteria and was comparable to antibiotics like penicillin in its germ-killing properties. Researcher Paul Belaiche reported his exhaustive studies of aromatherapy oils in his three-volume work *Traité de Phytothérapie et d'Aromathérapie* (Treatise on Phytotherapy and Aromatherapy). He tested the effectiveness of essential oils against specific bacteria. His findings on the effectiveness of oregano oil against many common and insidious bacteria were impressive. Belaiche found that oregano oil killed 96 percent of all pneumococcus bacteria; 92 percent of all neisseria, the bacteria responsible for gonorrhea and proteus meningitis; and 92 percent of staphylococcus bacteria, the culprit in some types of food poisoning. He also found that oregano oil eliminated 83 percent of streptococcus, which has been linked with strep throat, scarlet fever, rheumatic fever, and toxic shock syndrome, and 78 percent of enterococcus, which is linked with cystitis, wound infections, and anorexia.

What's more is that Belaiche's study also found that oregano oil killed 78 percent of candida bacteria, commonly linked with intestinal or systemic candida infections, and 78 percent of klebsiella bacteria, which has been linked to lung infections. (Check out Chapter 3 for more about candida.)

The *Journal of Food Protection* cites a study by researchers at the Department of Food Science at the University of Tennessee reporting impressive findings regarding oregano oil's potency against bacteria. Scientists found that oregano oil exhibited the most significant antibacterial action against common germs like staphylococcus, E. coli, and listeria. Researchers in the United Kingdom found that not only was oil of oregano effective against these common bacteria, it has antibacterial activity against 25 different bacteria. There are various potencies of oregano oil on the market. Some come in liquid form, while others come in gel capsules. Follow the dosage instructions on the label of the product you select. Because it is so powerful, oregano oil can also kill beneficial intestinal bacteria, so it is important to take probiotics while on any oregano oil regimen. Be sure to keep a two- to three-hour space between taking oregano oil and probiotics.

Broken Bones and Fractures

We often think of our bones as concrete-like structures that are static, nonliving, and noninteracting with the rest of our bodies. But this viewpoint is far from the truth. Bones are alive—like other tissue in our body. They are made up of living cells and are approximately 50 percent water. And unfortunately, it is not usually until they fracture or break that we think about the important role they play in maintaining the body's posture, balance, and immune system.

Our bones provide a constant supply of healthy blood to our organs and tissues. They act as mineral bank accounts for our bodies, storing excess minerals until they can be used by the body or excreted. Bones even assist with hormonal balance in our bodies.

Thanks to dairy advertising boards, we tend to think of bones as almost exclusively made up of calcium, which is inaccurate. Bones also comprise more than two dozen elements, such as phosphorus and magnesium. Bones are constantly being rebuilt by cells called osteoblasts and broken down by osteoclasts. When the breakdown of bones exceeds the rate of rebuilding, bones become weak. To use the bank account analogy again, if you always borrowed money from the bank and never repaid it, you would develop major credit problems and the bank would stop lending to you. The same applies to our bones: when we are always withdrawing minerals, but not depositing new ones, we deplete our bones' supply. When the bones become chronically depleted of minerals they become fragile and weak, and vulnerable to various types of illness and injuries.

Our bodies are made up of 206 bones, and any of them can be broken or fractured. A break occurs when the bone splits into more than one piece, while a fracture is a hairline crack that forms on the surface of the bone. Most breaks and fractures require the injured area to be immobilized, usually in a cast, to heal properly. In some situations surgery may be needed to pin the pieces of bone together. Fractures of the hip are most commonly the result of weakened, demineralized bones.

The Phytozyme Cure for Broken Bones and Fractures
The Diet

People suffering from a broken bone or fracture may be experiencing a deficiency in any or all of the enzymes needed to digest carbohydrates, fats, or proteins. If, after taking the quizzes in Chapter 4, you found that you were a Phytozyme Cure Carb, Fat, or Protein Type, follow the diet for that particular type. If you could not determine one clear type, follow the Phytozyme Cure Combination Type diet. If you've experienced broken bones or fractures more than once, you may wish to follow the dietary and supplement suggestions suggested under "Osteoporosis," as you may be experiencing bone demineralization.

Regardless which of the Phytozyme Cure Type diets you follow, emphasize foods that contain lycopene and hesperetin in your diet. See the chart "Phytonutrients: What They Do and Where to Find Them" on page 32 for more about these specific phytonutrients.

Despite what dairy board advertisements suggest, you cannot strengthen your bones simply by eating more dairy products. You need highly usable sources of calcium in your diet, including carrots and carrot juice (diluted 50:50 with water), kale, dark leafy greens, sesame seeds, tahini (sesame butter), broccoli, almonds, almond butter, kelp, oats, and navy beans. Kelp is an excellent choice, since it also provides many other minerals to help bones heal.

If you are experiencing menopause or are postmenopausal, you may need to address possible hormone imbalances to ensure proper bone healing. Balancing hormones in women is also imperative to bone health and healing, since estrogen and testosterone help the body to assimilate calcium and other bone-building minerals. The mineral boron acts as a mild estrogen replacement therapy in postmenopausal women who are deficient in this hormone and at risk of weakened bones. Yet, research shows that the average North American obtains only half the amount of boron necessary to prevent bone demineralization. Boron is found in greatest concentrations in fruit, particularly apples, dates, grapes, peaches, pears, and raisins. It is also found in legumes and nuts, especially almonds and hazelnuts, as well as in honey.

Supplementing the Diet

Supplementing your diet with a high-quality full-spectrum digestive enzyme formula that includes amylase, lipase, and protease, among other enzymes, is beneficial to helping your bones heal. Take 1 to 3 enzyme capsules or tablets with every meal to help your body break down the carbohydrates, fats, and proteins in your food into the natural sugars, essential fatty acids, and amino acids needed for optimal bone healing. Lipase is essential to carry calcium across the intestinal wall for your body to use, and protease carries calcium in the blood.

It can also be helpful to supplement with one or more of the following enzymes between meals on an empty stomach: bromelain, chymotrypsin, nattokinase, papain, protease, serrapeptidase, super-oxide dismutase (SOD), or trypsin, or a single product that includes some or all of these enzymes. Start with 1 capsule or tablet of your chosen enzyme(s) on an empty stomach 20 minutes before or at least 1 hour after meals, three times daily. You can gradually increase that amount to 3 capsules or tablets at a time, three times daily, or more with the guidance of a nutritional medicine practitioner experienced in systemic enzyme therapy.

You can supplement with the phytonutrient ipriflavone (7-isopropoxy-isoflavone) as well, because it inhibits the loss of bone cells. Working with other nutrients, it increases bone mineral density, stimulates bone cells, and increases calcium absorption.

Glucosamine sulfate is also important to bone health. It is an amino sugar that helps with bone formation. Take 1500 milligrams of glucosamine daily with meals.

To help speed bone healing and address any mineral deficiencies, you may need a mineral supplement. (There are many excellent products formulated specifically for bone health.) I've discussed calcium and boron, but here are other minerals to consider:

- *Magnesium* helps the body to absorb and utilize calcium.
- *Phosphorus* is important to bone mineralization and the synthesis of collagen, which is a glue-like protein that helps to hold everything together.
- *Potassium* enhances calcium absorption.
- *Silica* is required for bone collagen formation and healing bone fractures.
- *Zinc* is necessary for bone growth and development and works synergistically with calcium.

Numerous vitamins are essential to bone health and healing. Here are the most important ones:

- *Vitamin A* aids bone and teeth formation. Take 2500 to 5000 IU daily. If you're pregnant, lactating, or suffering from liver disease, avoid taking supplemental vitamin A unless you're under the guidance of a qualified health professional.
- *B vitamins* (6, 9, and 12) protect the body from a buildup of homocysteine—a protein by-product that interferes with collagen formation needed for bone development and health.

Take a 100-milligram B-complex supplement containing these
B vitamins.

- *Vitamin C* is essential to produce adequate levels of bone
  collagen.
- *Vitamin D3* draws calcium from the blood into the bones,
  stimulating the absorption of calcium from supplements and
  the diet to form stronger bones.
- *Vitamin K* is required for the production of osteocalcin (a bone
  protein), which provides structure to bone tissue and is critical
  to repair. Without it, bones become fragile and break easily.

Without adequate vitamins and minerals like those listed above,
the bones simply cannot properly absorb calcium. Fortunately, a
high-potency and high-quality vitamin and mineral supplement can
usually supply all of these vitamins and minerals.

Of course, while your break or fracture is healing, you need to
keep the area still. However, after you've healed, getting bone-building
exercise is important. Walking, rebounding, running, weight training,
and other impact or weight-bearing activities are best, provided your
bones are strong enough and have not been excessively depleted of
minerals or nutrients.

Cancer

We all have cancer cells in our body all the time. For most of us,
our bodies seek out and destroy these cells before they multiply to
form a tumor and damage healthy tissue. We have our immune systems, an important cell-regulating process called apoptosis, and an
amazing network of controls within the genetic material of our cells
to thank for this. But sometimes when the body's defenses aren't
strong enough, aren't adequately supported, or must deal with a high
volume of carcinogenic (cancer-causing) toxins, cancerous cells can
become out of control and attempt to infiltrate various organs and
tissues—a process known as metastasis. When this happens, a person

may be diagnosed with cancer. Be aware that cancer may also be diagnosed before metastasis occurs—for instance, in the case of a malignant tumor.

Known Risk Factors for Cancer

Age: Most cancers strike people who are over the age of 45. The link to aging may be the result of a lifetime of poor dietary and lifestyle choices, but not always. Younger people can also develop cancer.

Bad habits: Smoking, excessive alcohol consumption, and illicit drug use are all linked to cancer.

Geographical location: Industrialized countries have much higher rates of certain cancers than undeveloped countries. Environmental factors such as lifestyle, culture, diet, and water and air quality may explain this.

Environment: Being exposed to carcinogens can put a serious strain on your body's immune system, preventing it from fighting cancer cells. The most common carcinogens include cigarette smoke, pesticides, pollution, fragrances, and food additives.

Poor diet: High fat intake is linked to breast, colon, ovarian, kidney, lung, and endometrial cancers. Low fiber intake is linked to higher rates of colon cancer.

Inactivity: Sedentary lifestyles are linked with higher rates of many cancers.

Family history: Many people think that family genetics are the only factor for cancer. But family members share more than DNA; they may also share poor dietary choices, sedentary lifestyles, or other bad habits that make them more likely to get cancer.

Income: Lower income is linked to higher rates of stomach cancer, lung cancer (in men), cervical cancer, and cancers of the mouth, pharynx, larynx, and esophagus, while higher income is linked to higher incidence of skin cancer, breast cancer, prostate cancer, and colon cancer (in men). Because a lot of processed and packaged foods are relatively cheap to buy, many lower income individuals may not be eating healthy, natural foods.

Education: People with lower levels of education are linked to higher incidence of cancer and tend to have less access to cancer-prevention information. A lack of a formal education does not mean you must succumb to cancer. Regardless of your education level, stay informed. Read about cancer prevention strategies.

The Phytozyme Cure for Cancer
The Diet

Based on my clinical experience and research, I have found that most people suffering from cancer are eating more carbohydrates (usually in the form of sweets or sugary foods) or meat than their body can handle. To address these concerns, follow the Phytozyme Cure Carb Type or the Phytozyme Cure Protein Type diet outlined in Chapter 4.

Phytonutrients appear to work on different levels against cancer. Some speed the process of regulating damaged cells—apoptosis—while others boost the immune system, or protect the genetic material in the cells against damage. All of the processes are important in the prevention or treatment of cancer. Emphasize foods that contain alpha-carotene, astaxanthin, beta-sitosterol, chlorogenic acid, cryptoxanthin, curcumin, ellagic acid, ferulic acid, hesperetin, indole-3-carbinol, isoflavones, lycopene, naringin, perrillyl alcohol, proanthocyanidin, quercetin, resveratrol, saponins, silymarin, sulforaphane, tangeretin, terpene limonoids, and zeaxanthin in your diet. See the chart "Phytonutrients: What They Do and Where to Find Them" on page 32 for more about these specific phytonutrients.

It is important for people who have cancer to detoxify their diets, as well as boost their body's ability to detoxify itself to ensure maximum cellular functioning. Refer to Chapter 3 for more on how to get the harmful substances out of your diet. Pay particular attention to foods that are high in fat; foods that contain artificial substances like trans fats, hydrogenated fats, colors, and additives, since research is finding many of these ingredients are carcinogens; smoked foods; pickled foods; barbecued foods; and alcohol—all of which can play a harmful role in the development of cancer or which may contain carcinogens.

Research demonstrates that vegetarians have lower incidences of cancer. Your diet should be vegetarian or primarily vegetarian. Eat lots of vegetables, particularly leafy greens, whole grains, fruits, legumes, nuts, seeds, seaweed, and sea vegetables. (If you do choose meat products, choose only lean organic poultry and wild fish.)

Fiber also plays a critical role in the prevention of cancer. Not only does fiber help to keep us regular, certain types can actually bind to various types of toxins in our bodies to eliminate them in our stools and prevent them from doing damage to our bodily tissues. Fortunately, if you emphasize vegetables, beans, and whole grains in your diet, as recommended in Chapter 4, you'll automatically be eating more fiber.

Top 12 Cancer-Fighting Foods   As you can see from the list of anti-cancer phytonutrients and the chart of their food sources on page 32, there are many foods that help to prevent and fight cancer. Here are some excellent choices:

- **Apples:** An apple a day really might keep the doctor away when it comes to cancer. Research shows that an apple a day lowers a woman's risk of breast cancer by 29 percent.7 Be sure to choose organic apples, since conventionally grown apples are typically heavily sprayed with pesticides, some of which can be linked to cancer.

- **Broccoli** and **broccoli sprouts:** Both broccoli and broccoli sprouts contain the phytonutrient sulforaphane, which promotes the production of anticancer enzymes. Broccoli and broccoli sprouts also contain isothiocyanates and indole-3-carbinol—phytonutrients which help prevent the growth of tumors.

- **Brussels sprouts:** These underrated veggies contain the phyto-nutrients indoles, compounds that can stop uncontrolled cell growth linked to cancer.

- **Carrots:** The phytonutrient beta-carotene (as well as other carotenes) found in carrots reduces excessive estrogen in breast tissue that can lead to tumor growth.

- **Chilies:** Capsaicin is a potent anti-inflammatory phytonutrient found in chilies, which appears to kill cancer cells.

- **Eggs:** In recent studies, women with the highest doses of choline—a nutrient found in eggs that is necessary for proper cell functioning—were 24 percent less likely to develop breast cancer compared to women who had low levels of choline in their diet.[8]

- **Garlic:** Sulfur compounds in garlic may prevent cancerous tumors from growing.

- **Green tea:** More and more research touts the cancer-defying properties of green tea. Green tea contains the phytonutrient epigallocatechin gallate (EGCG), which starves cancerous cells by shutting down the blood supply that feeds them and cancerous tumors. It also reduces overproduction of the hormone estradiol, a form of estrogen that is linked to estrogen-related cancers like breast cancer.

- **Lemons:** These citrus nutritional powerhouses contain more than 20 anticancer components and help to balance body chemistry—acidic tissues and bodily fluids may be a risk factor for cancer. Simply squeeze fresh lemon into pure water or green tea daily.

- **Mushrooms:** Mushrooms offer tremendous protection against cancer and can intervene at most stages of cancer progression. But don't choose garden-variety button mush-rooms. For their medicinal effects, try more exotic varieties.

If you can't find them fresh, you can choose to take them in tincture or capsule form. *Cordyceps* mushrooms are available in supplement form and are helpful for rebuilding a person's energy and strength when dealing with cancer or other health conditions. *Maitake D-fraction* mushroom extract helps to stimulate apoptosis (cancer cell death), particularly in prostate cancer (where they have a 90 percent cancer cell kill rate). They can also reduce the side effects of chemotherapy and radiation. *Reishi* mushrooms help to eliminate carcinogens from the body, while protecting against bacterial and viral infections, including those that may result from a radiation- or chemotherapy-depleted immune system. *Royal agaricus* mushrooms contain beta glucan, a natural immune booster that also stimulates the body's natural killer cells. *Shiitake* mushrooms tend to be available in most grocery stores, which is great because they contain a phytonutrient called lentinan, which appears to slow tumor growth.[9]

- **Olive oil:** Extra-virgin olive oil contains oleic acid, an antioxidant that has been proven to kill cancer cells on contact. This nutrient may also render breast cancer genes inactive. It is quite easy to get olive oil into your diet by making it the main ingredient in salad dressings. The ratio of oil to acid (vinegar or lemon juice) in a dressing is 3:1—for example, 3 parts olive oil to 1 part balsamic vinegar. Simply add some fresh or dried herbs, berries, a touch of maple syrup, or other flavorful ingredient and shake or blend for a delicious homemade salad dressing that's ready in minutes.

Supplementing the Diet

Supplementing your diet with a high-quality full-spectrum digestive enzyme formula that includes amylase, lipase, and protease, among other enzymes, is also beneficial for cancer sufferers. Take 1 to 3 enzyme capsules or tablets with every meal to help your body break down the carbohydrates, fats, and proteins in your food into the natural sugars, essential fatty acids, and amino acids needed for optimal healing.

You can also supplement with one or more of the following enzymes between meals on an empty stomach: bromelain, chymotrypsin, protease, serrapeptidase, superoxide dismutase (SOD), or trypsin, or a single product that includes some or all of these enzymes; these enzymes can be helpful for various types of cancer. Start with 5 capsules or tablets of your chosen enzyme(s) on an empty stomach 20 minutes before or at least 1 hour after meals, three times daily. You can gradually increase that amount to 10 capsules or tablets at a time, three times daily, or more with the guidance of a nutritional medicine practitioner experienced in systemic enzyme therapy. If you are experiencing cancer, I strongly encourage you to work with a holistic health practitioner who is well versed in systemic enzyme therapy and its use in cancer.

Enzyme therapy really shines when it comes to cancer. Not only do enzymes help improve the immune response, they can chemically alter tumor by-products to make them less damaging to the body and even change the surface of the tumor cells to help the body to recognize them as cancer cells and destroy them.

Supplement with additional nutrients, particularly those that strengthen the immune system (vitamins A, C, and E, and beta-carotene, zinc, copper, folic acid, riboflavin, pyridoxine, and pantothenic acid), neutralize carcinogens (vitamins A and C, selenomethionine, and L-cysteine), and prevent cellular and DNA damage (vitamins A, C, and E, beta carotene, selenium, zinc, and manganese). You can get most of these nutrients from a high-quality multivitamin.

Higher doses of beta-carotene and vitamins A, C, D, and E are showing increasing promise in inhibiting diseases like cancer. I normally recommend 10,000 IU of vitamin A, 5000 to 10,000 milligrams of vitamin C in 2000-milligram doses spread throughout the day or until you reach bowel tolerance (you'll know when you experience loose stools), 4000 IU of vitamin D, and 800 IU of vitamin E for the treatment of cancer. Do not take high doses of beta-carotene if you are a smoker with cancer.

I also recommend 455 milligrams of choline daily, particularly for breast cancer and breast cancer prevention.

Chronic Fatigue Syndrome

Chronic fatigue syndrome (CFS) is a serious disease. It comprises a range of debilitating symptoms that limit a person's capacity to do everyday things that most of us take for granted. It can be characterized by not only oppressive fatigue but also overwhelming weakness, body and joint pain, and mental exhaustion. Needless to say, CFS is a disease that can disrupt quality of life.

Research has linked CFS to damage of the blood-brain barrier, which can be caused by infection, inflammation, or stress, or may be the result of genetic predisposition. When this barrier is compromised, it is easier for other toxins and harmful chemicals to reach the brain and wreak havoc.

Fatigue and body pain do not necessarily mean a person has CFS—these symptoms can be attributed to many health conditions. A proper diagnosis from an informed medical doctor is required to rule out other disorders, such as AIDS, anemia, hypothyroidism, or mononucleosis, and to obtain a diagnosis of CFS.

The Phytozyme Cure for Chronic Fatigue Syndrome
The Diet
People suffering from chronic fatigue syndrome can be experiencing a deficiency in any or all of the enzymes needed to digest carbohydrates, fats, or proteins. If, after taking the quizzes in Chapter 4, you found that you were a Phytozyme Cure Carb, Fat, or Protein Type, follow the diet for that particular type. If you could not determine one clear type, follow the Phytozyme Cure Combination Type diet.

Emphasize foods that contain anthocyanins, astaxanthin, catechins, curcumin, ellagic acid, hesperetin, lipoic acid, naringin, pectin, proanthocyanidin, resveratrol, silymarin, sulforaphane, tangeretin, tannins, terpene limonoids, and zeaxanthin in your diet. See the chart "Phytonutrients: What They Do and Where to Find Them" on page 32 for more about these specific phytonutrients.

People managing CFS must be as conscious of what they don't eat as what they do eat. Many CFS sufferers have undiagnosed food allergies or sensitivities to gluten and dairy products. If you have CFS, you should also avoid processed and packaged foods, which often contain preservatives, colors, additives, and excessive sugars.

Supplementing the Diet

Supplementing your diet with a high-quality full-spectrum digestive enzyme formula that includes amylase, lipase, and protease, among other enzymes, is also beneficial. Take 1 to 3 enzyme capsules or tablets with every meal to help your body break down the carbohydrates, fats, and proteins in your food into the natural sugars, essential fatty acids, and amino acids needed for optimal healing.

It can also be helpful to supplement with one or more of the following enzymes between meals on an empty stomach: bromelain, cellulose, chymotrypsin, protease, serrapeptidase, superoxide dismutase (SOD), or trypsin, or a single product that includes some or all of these enzymes. Start with 3 capsules or tablets of your chosen enzyme(s) on an empty stomach 20 minutes before or at least 1 hour after meals, three times daily. You can gradually increase that amount to 5 capsules or tablets at a time, three times daily, or more with the guidance of a nutritional medicine practitioner experienced in systemic enzyme therapy.

There are a number of other nutritional supplements that can improve or relieve the symptoms of chronic fatigue syndrome. Research has demonstrated that many people diagnosed with CFS are deficient in magnesium, which is needed for energy production at the cellular level. Many vitamins, and B vitamins in particular, are also needed for energy production. They work together, making a B-complex vitamin combined with extra vitamin B12 an important energy booster. Take a high-quality multivitamin and mineral, along with an additional 100-milligram B-complex supplement. Additional magnesium totaling 1000 milligrams may be necessary.

The same can be said of coenzyme Q10 (CoQ10) which is also needed for manufacturing energy at the cellular level. Take 100 to 300 milligrams of CoQ10 daily.

People with CFS often have digestive problems. A high-quality probiotic supplement can be beneficial to help control candida and overgrowth of harmful intestinal bacteria. Probiotics work most effectively when taken on an empty stomach at night or in the morning.

Supporting brain health is critical, and daily consumption of fish oils provide essential fatty acids that support nerve and brain function, including the blood-brain barrier I explained earlier. For more information, consult my book *The Brain Wash*.

CFS sufferers can also benefit from the energy-building effects of Siberian ginseng and the antiviral natural powerhouse wild oregano oil. Follow dosage instructions on the package of the products you choose. Because it is so powerful, oregano oil can also kill beneficial intestinal bacteria, so it is important to take probiotics along with any oregano oil regimen, with a two- to three-hour space between them.

Colitis and Crohn's Disease

Both colitis and Crohn's disease are digestive disorders in which the intestinal lining becomes inflamed. Colitis sufferers experience painful inflammation in parts of the colon; for those with Crohn's disease, the entire digestive tract can be inflamed (from the mouth to the rectum). In some cases of both conditions, ulcerations may form in the affected areas.

Symptoms of these conditions include weakness, fatigue, lethargy, diarrhea alternating with constipation, abdominal pain, fever, hemorrhoids, dehydration, mineral loss, weight loss, and blood in the stools.

The medical community has not yet pinpointed a single cause for either of these conditions. However, there are many factors that may play a role, including poor food choices, chronic stress, genetics, nutritional deficiencies, and bowel flora imbalances, among others. Since the drug treatment options for colitis and Crohn's disease have severe side effects and long-term health implications, natural medicine can be particularly helpful.

The Phytozyme Cure for Colitis and Crohn's Disease
The Diet

Most people suffering from colitis or Crohn's disease are eating more carbohydrates—sugary foods, milk sugars, or gluten-containing grains—than their body can handle. To address these concerns, follow the Phytozyme Cure Carb Type diet outlined in Chapter 4.

Emphasize foods that contain anthocyanin, astaxanthin, beta-sitosterol, catechins, curcumin, hesperetin, quercetin, resveratrol, saponins, silymarin, and tannins in your diet. See the chart "Phytonutrients: What They Do and Where to Find Them" on page 32 for more about these specific phytonutrients.

While colitis and Crohn's can be linked to an intestinal infection or stress, diet usually plays a major role, in the form of food sensitivities or allergies, or poor dietary choices. The major culprits are wheat, gluten, dairy products, corn, and eggs. The symptoms of lactose intolerance (a reaction to the sugar in dairy products) can mimic the symptoms of colitis or Crohn's disease. It is important to avoid all of these foods and gluten-containing grains and foods made with them, including pasta, bread, pastries, cookies, cakes.

Consumption of processed and sugar-laden foods, and a lack of dietary enzymes and fiber, can contribute significantly to both conditions. It is essential to eliminate the harmful food substances we discussed in Chapter 3 (food additives, sugar, artificial sweeteners and sorbitol, dairy, and fried foods). In addition, avoid coffee and caffeine, carbonated beverages, citrus fruit, nuts, and seeds. It is important to very gradually increase the fiber in your diet and be sure you're drinking 8 cups of water per day.

Freshly made vegetable juices are helpful for colitis and Crohn's disease sufferers. They contain a large number of nutrients and phytonutrients, which aid healing and stave off the nutrient deficiencies that are common with these conditions. Be sure to dilute any juices with water to a 50:50 ratio since juices are high in sugars.

Supplementing the Diet

Probiotics are essential for the Crohn's disease or colitis sufferer, and you can find out more information about them in Chapter 4. Take probiotics as directed on the package, on an empty stomach either first thing in the morning or before bed.

Phytozyme therapy can make a big difference in these two illnesses. Enzymes can help normalize digestion, conquer infection, and lessen inflammation. Phytonutrients can assist healing of the intestinal wall. Supplementing your diet with a high-quality full-spectrum digestive enzyme formula that includes amylase, lipase, and protease, among other enzymes, is also beneficial. Take 1 to 3 enzyme capsules or tablets with every meal to help your body break down the carbohydrates, fats, and proteins in your food into the natural sugars, essential fatty acids, and amino acids needed for optimal healing.

It can also be helpful to supplement with one or more of the following enzymes between meals on an empty stomach: bromelain, papain, protease, serrapeptidase, superoxide dismutase (SOD), or trypsin, or a single product that includes some or all of these enzymes. Start with 1 capsule or tablet of your chosen enzyme(s) on an empty stomach 20 minutes before or at least 1 hour after meals, three times daily. You can gradually increase that amount to 3 capsules or tablets at a time, three times daily, or more with the guidance of a nutritional medicine practitioner experienced in systemic enzyme therapy.

More specifically, you can take 1500 milligrams of bromelain daily and 400 milligrams of protease on an empty stomach to lessen inflammation. Reduce this dosage if it aggravates your symptoms. Papain is also helpful for reducing inflammation. Take 1500 milligrams between meals on an empty stomach.

Supplementary turmeric and quercetin can help with food sensitivities. Take 1 to 3 grams of turmeric powder daily or 400 to 600 milligrams of curcumin (the standardized extract of turmeric) daily, and 1000 milligrams of quercetin per day with meals.

The amino acid glutamine (also known as L-glutamine) has been shown in research to be as effective as the drug prednisone in managing Crohn's disease, making it an excellent supplement to include in your program.

Vitamin C is helpful to lessen inflammation and deal with any food sensitivities. Take 500 to 1000 milligrams at a time, three times daily.

Research suggests that fish oil might be beneficial to colitis and Crohn's disease patients. In a study in the *New England Journal of Medicine,* 59 percent of Crohn's disease patients taking fish oil capsules stayed symptom-free, compared to 26 percent given placebos. In another study, colitis patients taking fish oil showed less evidence of inflammation and felt better than patients who took a placebo. They were also able to gain weight and cut back on steroid drugs.

In my practice, I've seen some great healing results with herbs, which can also help soothe the intestinal walls. My preferred choices include aloe vera juice and slippery elm. Take 1 ounce of aloe vera juice in the morning on an empty stomach. Take 1 teaspoon of slippery elm in 1 cup of boiling water, three times daily. Alternatively, take 6 slippery elm lozenges, one at a time, throughout the day. They are available in many health food stores.

Depression

Everyone feels down at some point, usually as a reaction to difficult circumstances. For the purpose of this book, however, I am referring to diagnosed clinical depression. In such cases, the person experiences a prolonged sadness that is out of proportion with the apparent cause. The physical and psychological symptoms affect a person's capacity to function normally in the world.

Depression is often accompanied by sleep disruption, fatigue, anxiety, mood swings, prolonged lapses of concentration, pain, apathy, decreased sex drive, and suicidal thoughts. Because these symptoms can be attributed to other diseases or conditions, it is always important to consult a medical doctor for a diagnosis.

While this section is about clinical depression, the suggestions I present will do wonders for treating the symptoms of other emotional imbalances (sadness, mood swings, anxiety) as well.

The Phytozyme Cure for Depression
The Diet
Poor nutrition, in my opinion, is one of the greatest causes of depression, and one of the easiest and most overlooked solutions. My clinical experience tells me that depression cannot be managed in the long term without addressing the diet.

Poor diet is frequently linked to depression because food additives, chemicals, alcohol, sugar, and sugar substitutes can have severely negative effects on our mental and physical health. Combined with the side effects of both pharmaceutical medications and recreational drugs, consuming these substances will biochemically depress the proper functioning of our bodies and minds. Eating a healthful diet helps the body balance hormone levels, including important brain hormones that help us feel good. For example, complex carbohydrates from vegetables, legumes, and whole grains help the brain manufacture serotonin, a "feel good" neurotransmitter that is needed to prevent depression.

From my clinical experience and research, I have found that most people suffering from depression are eating more carbohydrates, usually in the form of sugars, than their body can handle. To address this concern, follow the Phytozyme Cure Carb Type diet in Chapter 4 and be sure to eliminate the harmful foods outlined in Chapter 3 (such as sugar and food additives like MSG).

Also, emphasize foods that contain astaxanthin, catechins, curcumin, lipoic acid, naringin, proanthocyanidin, resveratrol, and tangeretin in your diet. See the chart "Phytonutrients: What They Do and Where to Find Them" on page 32 for more about these specific phytonutrients.

It's also important to address possible food allergens, which can be tough to pinpoint. The most common ones are dairy, wheat, gluten, MSG, sugars, artificial sweeteners, and food colors. Removing these foods from the diet in favor of wholesome, nutrient-dense food choices frequently improves mood.

Many of my depressive clients confirm that they are in the habit of skipping meals (like breakfast) or waiting long periods of time between eating. This confirms a suspicion that blood sugar imbalances may be a factor in depression. Keep blood sugar levels balanced by eating a healthy snack or meal every two to three hours.

Flaxseed oil can also help treat depression. Take 2 tablespoons daily. You can pour it over baked sweet potatoes or vegetables, or blend some into a smoothie.

Supplementing the Diet

Supplementing your diet with a high-quality full-spectrum digestive enzyme formula that includes the amylase, invertase, lactase, maltose, lipase, and protease enzymes is beneficial. Take 1 to 3 enzyme capsules or tablets with every meal to help your body break down the carbohydrates, fats, and proteins in your food into the natural sugars, essential fatty acids, and amino acids needed for optimal healing.

In addition to healthy food, supplements such as 5-HTP, Saint-John's-wort, and ginkgo biloba are effective in reducing symptoms of depression. As a precursor to serotonin, 5-HTP helps to restore healthy levels of this much-needed brain chemical. I recommend taking 50 to 100 milligrams of 5-HTP at bedtime for 2 months. Despite one well-publicized study that demonstrated the ineffectiveness of Saint-John's-wort against severe depression, countless research studies show that it is effective against mild and moderate depression, and it also helps raise serotonin levels in the brain. I recommend

900 to 1200 milligrams daily. However, avoid taking Saint-John's-wort if you are taking pharmaceutical antidepressants, and do not take it within two to three hours of sunlight exposure. As for ginkgo biloba, it helps bring more oxygen to the brain through the blood stream, and your brain needs oxygen to work properly. Take 60 milligrams three times daily.

Because so many vitamins and minerals are involved with mood balancing, it is important that you address any possible deficiencies by taking a high-quality multivitamin and mineral supplement with meals. In addition, because the B-complex vitamins are so vital for restoring balanced moods, take an extra 100-milligram B-complex supplement daily.

Essential fatty acids are necessary to treat depression, as they are required to create healthy brain cells and are involved in regulating neurotransmitters—the brain hormones that balance mood. Take 3000 milligrams daily of either fish or flaxseed oil, or 500 milligrams of DHA or EPA, or a blend of both.

S-adenosylmethionine (SAMe) occurs naturally in the body and helps regulate certain biochemical reactions, including those linked to mood regulation. Take 400 to 1600 milligrams daily of SAMe to ensure your brain can make important mood elevating hormones.

Supplementing with 2000 to 4000 IU of vitamin D daily can help with depression, because it helps the body make serotonin.

People suffering from depression should also supplement their daily routines through more fresh air and physical activity. Exercise is a natural antidepressant, and engaging in regular cardiovascular exercise like brisk walking or jogging is good for your body and mind. And as always, drink lots of pure water to avoid dehydration.

Diabetes

Diabetes is a serious chronic health condition that is the result of elevated blood sugar levels. When blood sugar levels are too high, they become toxic to the organs, including the brain. Remember that our bodies need some sugar to provide energy for many functions. In diabetics, there can be two main problems with the way the body handles sugar. One is that the body has an insulin deficiency, which is the hormone your body needs to process sugar. The other problem is that the body's cells may be resistant to insulin, which prevents blood sugar from entering cells.

There are three types of diabetes: type 1, type 2, and gestational diabetes. While there are some variations in the three types, they are all serious medical conditions that need to be treated by a physician.

Type 1 is also called juvenile diabetes, since it usually develops in childhood or adolescence. Type 1 sufferers have severe insulin deficiencies and require insulin injections. Type 2 diabetes is also called adult-onset diabetes or non-insulin dependent diabetes. While this type usually strikes adults, it can also affect children. Type 2 is usually linked to eating too-high amounts of refined carbohydrates and sugars, being sedentary, and carrying excess weight. However, it is also the type that responds best to dietary and lifestyle changes. Gestational diabetes occurs in some women during pregnancy due to hormonal imbalances. Although it usually disappears after the baby is born, it still needs to be addressed because unregulated blood sugars may be damaging to the fetus.

Symptoms of diabetes include fatigue, insatiable thirst, frequent urination, excessive appetite, weight loss or gain, blurred vision, and irritability.

The Phytozyme Cure for Diabetes
The Diet
Most people suffering from diabetes are eating more carbohydrates or fats than their body can handle. To address these concerns, follow the Phytozyme Cure Carbohydrate Type or the Phytozyme Cure Fat Type dietary suggestions, depending on your Phytozyme Cure Type quiz results from Chapter 4.

Emphasize foods that contain alpha-carotene, anthocyanin, astaxanthin, beta carotene, catechins, chlorogenic acid, curcumin, ferulic acid, hesperetin, lipoic acid, lutein, naringin, resveratrol, and rutin in your diet. See the chart "Phytonutrients: What They Do and Where to Find Them" on page 32 for more about these specific phytonutrients.

Make vegetables the focal point of every meal. You should keep fruit consumption to a minimum; however, eating fruit is better than eating other types of sweets, provided that fruit is allowed by your physician.

Permanently adopting a healthy diet is the best thing a diabetic can do for his or her health. Be sure to eliminate the harmful substances in your diet, particularly refined carbohydrates and sugars, which include so-called healthy sweeteners like honey, maple sugar, and agave. Avoid "diet" and "sugar-free" products as well, because they typically contain synthetic sweeteners that are toxic to the body and damaging to diabetics and non-diabetics alike. (For more bad news on artificial sweeteners, see Chapter 3.) Instead, sweeten food with stevia.

Eat a diet high in fiber. Fiber helps to regulate blood sugar by keeping blood levels stable for long periods of time. A high-fiber diet also lowers cholesterol and triglycerides.

Add chromium-rich foods (I explain the benefits of chromium in Chapter 3) to your diet, including whole grains, eggs, shiitake mushrooms, liver, onions, garlic, cucumbers, green and yellow beans, and moderate amounts of fruit (if permitted by your doctor). Try to eat wild salmon twice a week or supplement with essential fatty acids (see below). Also, every day eat at least one large green salad with cold-pressed flaxseed oil dressing.

Supplementing the Diet

For diabetics, supplementing the diet with a high quality full-spectrum digestive enzyme formula that includes amylase, lipase, and protease, among other enzymes, is beneficial. Take 1 to 3 enzyme capsules or tablets with every meal to help your body break down the carbohydrates, fats, and proteins in your food into the natural sugars, essential fatty acids, and amino acids needed for optimal healing.

Between meals on an empty stomach, it can also be helpful to supplement with one or more of the following enzymes: bromelain, protease, serrapeptidase, superoxide dismutase (SOD), or trypsin, or a single product that includes some or all of these enzymes. Start with one capsule or tablet of your chosen enzyme(s) on an empty stomach 20 minutes before or at least one hour after meals, three times daily. You can gradually increase that amount to three capsules or tablets at a time, three times daily, or more with the guidance of a nutritional medicine practitioner who is experienced in systemic enzyme therapy.

Mineral supplements are also good for treating diabetes. Some studies link a deficiency of chromium, a mineral involved in blood sugar balance, with diabetes. (I tell you more about chromium in Chapter 3). Take 200 micrograms daily of either GTF chromium or chromium picolinate. The mineral vanadium helps the body use insulin more effectively, and I recommend a daily supplement of 25 micrograms.

Diabetics can also benefit from the following supplements:

Alpha lipoic, 300 milligrams daily, has powerful antioxidant properties to help heal the free radical damage involved in diabetes.

Bitter melon, 250 to 500 milligrams daily of a 10:1 extract, which can be beneficial for managing blood sugar. Do not take bitter melon if you are pregnant or nursing or are on insulin.

Coenzyme Q10, 100 to 200 milligrams daily, is also helpful for diabetes. CoQ10 is required for the proper functioning of every cell in your body.

Gymnema sylvestre extract, 400 milligrams daily, helps repair the pancreas, kidneys and liver—the organs that can be impaired by diabetes.

Omega-3 fatty acids, 3000 milligrams daily of fish or flaxseed oil, or 500 milligrams daily of DHA-EPA can help to counter inflammation, a causative factor for diabetes.

For additional information, read the section on homocysteine under "Heart Disease" on page 209, since high homocysteine levels have been implicated in diabetes.

Digestive Disorders

Professor Charles T. Copeland said, "To eat is human, to digest divine." When we suffer from digestive troubles such as bloating, indigestion, or discomfort, the importance of digestion and eating to maintaining harmony in our bodies becomes obvious. While there are many types of digestive problems, I find that the overall approach to treating them is mostly the same.

The Phytozyme Cure for Digestive Disorders
The Diet
Most people suffering from digestive disorders are eating more carbohydrates or fats than their body can handle. To address these concerns, follow the Phytozyme Cure Carb Type or the Phytozyme Cure Fat Type diet, depending on your quiz results from chapter 4.

Emphasize foods that contain anthocyanin, capsaicin, catechins, chlorogenic acid, curcumin, ellagic acid, hesperetin, quercetin, resveratrol, silymarin, tannins, and terpene limonoids in your diet. See the chart "Phytonutrients: What They Do and Where to Find Them" on page 32 for more about these specific phytonutrients.

Supplementing the Diet
Supplementing your diet with a high-quality full-spectrum digestive enzyme formula that includes the amylase, lipase, and protease enzymes is beneficial. Take 1 to 3 enzyme capsules or tablets with every meal to help your body break down the carbohydrates, fats, and proteins in your food into the natural sugars, essential fatty acids, and amino acids needed for optimal healing.

It can also be helpful to supplement with one or more of the following enzymes between meals on an empty stomach: alpha galactosidase, beta glucanase, bromelain, chymotrypsin, mucolase, serrapeptidase, superoxide dismutase (SOD), or trypsin, or a single product like Wobenzym N that includes some or all of these enzymes. Start by taking one capsule or tablet of your chosen enzyme(s) on an empty stomach 20 minutes before or at least 1 hour after meals, three times daily. You can gradually increase that amount to 3 capsules or tablets at a time, three times daily, or more with the guidance of a nutritional medicine practitioner who is experienced in systemic enzyme therapy.

In addition to the dietary and supplement suggestions I provide above, here are suggestions for particular digestive concerns you may have.

Appetite (Excessive)   I usually find that excessive appetite can be linked to insufficient nutrient intake or a parasite infection. A person is actually hungry for more *nutrients,* not necessarily more *food.* So if you are constantly hungry, you are probably malnourished; that is, your body is deficient in key nutrients. Switch to a healthier diet and your appetite will lessen.

There are two main herbs that act as appetite suppressants: thyme and fennel. You can make these herbs into a tea by allowing 1/2 teaspoon each of dried thyme and fennel to steep in boiled water for 5 minutes. Or, take supplements of these herbs by following directions on the label. Wheatgrass juice is also an effective appetite suppressant, since it is very nutrient dense.

To address a possible parasite infestation, take 2 wild oregano oil gel capsules three times daily and take 2 probiotic capsules nightly before bed on an empty stomach. I assume throughout *The Phytozyme Cure* that you have seen a physician to diagnose your health conditions. Similarly, if you suspect a parasite infestation, you should see a doctor.

Constipation   Characterized by infrequent bowel movements, hard stools, and abdominal bloating, constipation is a condition that many people experience at some point. However, for some, it is an ongoing problem.

Most people are shocked to learn constipation is less than three large bowel movements daily, so I provide some suggestions to help you become and stay regular.

Take 2000 milligrams of vitamin C three to five times daily, until you experience loose bowel movements, and then cut back to 2000 milligrams daily.

Once a day, you may also take psyllium *(Plantago ovata)* by mixing 2 teaspoons in an 8-ounce glass of water or juice (without sweeteners). Stir the mixture well, drink it, and drink another glass of water. Or add 2 teaspoons of flaxseed to a shake or cereal.

Eat a high-fiber diet including brown rice, fresh fruits, and plentiful amounts of vegetables. Drink 8 to 10 cups of pure water daily, since water is essential to keep your bowels moving. Squeeze the juice of half a lemon into hot water and drink first thing in the morning on an empty stomach (wait 1/2 hour before eating). The fresh juices of celery, apple, carrot, rhubarb, and spinach act as laxatives and can replace some, but not all, of your water intake. To avoid getting too much sugar, always dilute juices with water using a 50:50 ratio.

Take 2 capsules of probiotics nightly before bed on an empty stomach to ease constipation. Drink licorice root tea, since it is an effective bowel stimulant, and eat more magnesium-rich foods, such as nuts, whole grains, soy, and seafood.

Exercise several times per week, since exercise helps to keep your bowels moving.

Diarrhea If you experience loose bowel movements for more than a day or two, you should know this information about how to curb diarrhea.

The homeopathic remedy Arsenicum album is particularly effective for diarrhea that causes burning pain in the digestive tract and is accompanied by anxiety. The person may be thirsty for frequent small sips of water. Podophyllum is also helpful, particularly for profuse diarrhea with loud gas. Try taking the suitable remedy in a 30X potency every 2 hours.

Herbs like agrimony (steep 1 teaspoon of dried leaves in 1 cup of boiling water for 10 minutes and take 1 to 3 cups per day), blackberry and raspberry leaves (steep 2 teaspoons of dried herb in boiling water), and peppermint (steep 1 to 2 teaspoons of dried herb in boiling water). Peppermint has an antispasmodic action on the intestines.

If you suspect that pathogens may be a cause of diarrhea, take 2 gel capsules of wild oregano oil three times daily to help fight them. Also, take 2 probiotic capsules nightly before bed on an empty stomach to get good-bacteria benefits.

Since diarrhea can put you at risk of dehydration, be sure to drink plenty of liquids, including herbal teas, water, or a broth made from boiled potatoes with some Celtic sea salt (this type of salt is high in sodium, potassium, and other minerals to replace lost minerals).

Eat cooked fruits like applesauce and cooked carrots. Also, eat plenty of raw apples, because the fiber in apples (pectin) provides bulk to watery stools. Just be sure to avoid apple juice, because it tends to have the opposite effect.

And remember that food sensitivities likely play a role in diarrhea, so I recommend that you avoid the foods that most commonly cause digestive problems for many people, particularly wheat, dairy products, and gluten. Eliminate them from your diet for a few months and see if your condition improves.

Flatulence   Flatulence, also known simply as "gas," can be a physically uncomfortable and personally embarrassing problem. Luckily, herbs like aniseed, dill, caraway, parsley, fennel, and ginger are great remedies for flatulence. Aniseed is proven in human studies to dispel gas. Take up to 3 cups of tea per day (steep 1/2 teaspoon of dried, crushed seeds in 1 cup of boiling water for 5 to 10 minutes). Fennel dispels gas and eases bloating and digestive spasms (simmer 1 teaspoon of crushed seeds in 1 cup of boiling water for 10 to 15 minutes). Ginger not only dispels gas but helps to quell nausea, increases bile secretion, and tones the bowel. Add 1/2 inch to 1 inch of fresh gingerroot while juicing carrots or apples.

Since gas is caused by intestinal bacteria that ferment in the colon, take 2 capsules of probiotics nightly before bed on an empty stomach.

Do not drink liquids 30 minutes before or after eating, since the excess liquid can cause food to putrefy and cause poor digestion. You should also avoid carbonated beverages, as they introduce excess gas into your system.

If legumes or vegetables are the culprits of flatulence, be sure to take an enzyme formula that includes alpha galactosidase and beta galactosidase with every meal to help digest the fiber contained in these foods.

Also, eat small amounts of fruit and only on an empty stomach, because its high sugar content can contribute to bacterial imbalances.

Gastric Ulcers Gastric ulcers are holes in the lining of the stomach. Licorice root is effective for gastric ulcers and studies show that it actually accelerates their healing. Use a tablet or capsule form of deglycyrrhizinated licorice (DGL), since it is effective but does not upset the body's sodium-potassium balance. Follow package instructions to determine the right amount to take.

Aloe vera juice is a proven therapy to heal inflamed intestinal walls and ulcers. Take 1 ounce on an empty stomach upon rising.

A medical study showed that drinking cabbage juice regularly can heal ulcerations. The amino acid L-glutamine, which is found in cabbage, works by nourishing the cells that line the stomach and esophagus so they can repair themselves. Cabbage juice also contains cancer-preventing agents called glucosinolates. You might try making your own fresh cabbage juice using a juicer, or blending cabbage with water, straining, then drinking the mixture. I'll warn you that it doesn't taste great on its own, but you can add an apple to the juicer or blender to make it more palatable.

Take 2 capsules of probiotics nightly before bed on an empty stomach.

Heartburn or Indigestion Anyone who has suffered from heartburn or indigestion knows that the characteristic burning sensation in the esophagus is not only uncomfortable but may even be painful. Although we often think that having too much stomach acid is the cause of these conditions, ironically, heartburn and indigestion are usually caused by having insufficient stomach acid to digest your food.

To simplify digestion, stick to small, frequent meals throughout the day. Avoid fried foods, hydrogenated fats (like margarine), or heated oils, including those that are heated during processing (which is almost all oils found in grocery stores, so opt for cold-pressed oils from your local health food store). Do not drink any liquids with your meals (or within 1/2 hour before or 1 hour after meals) so you do not dilute digestive enzymes and they can do their work, and cut back on meat, coffee, tea, white sugar, and alcohol consumption. I recommend that you do not lie down directly after meals.

Licorice root and aloe vera juice are great for easing heartburn. Use deglycyrrhizinated licorice (DGL), since it is effective but does not upset the body's sodium-potassium balance. Follow package instructions. Also, take 1 ounce of aloe vera juice on an empty stomach upon rising.

While it may be tempting to pop antacid pills, they have long-term damaging effects such as acid rebound. Plus they contain aluminum, which research links to many serious health conditions (see my book *The Brain Wash* for more information).

Along with these suggestions, take a multivitamin and mineral supplement daily (many nutrients are required for the body to make sufficient stomach acid), and you'll likely experience dramatic improvements.

Irritable Bowel Syndrome   Follow the Phytozyme Cure Carb Type Diet and see the additional information found under "Colitis and Crohn's Disease" on page 179.

Precancerous Stomach Lesions   Similar in symptoms to ulcers, precancerous stomach lesions are typically diagnosed through a biopsy. If you suspect ulcers or lesions due to a sudden loss of appetite or weight, you should see a doctor immediately to rule out cancer or a precancerous condition.

Numerous studies demonstrate the effectiveness of beta-carotene or vitamin C to prevent precancerous stomach lesions from becoming cancerous. I recommend you supplement your diet with 2000 milligrams of vitamin C and beta-carotene. However, avoid beta-carotene if you are a smoker, since research shows the combination may accelerate cancer.

Aloe vera juice is a proven therapy to heal inflamed intestinal walls and lesions. Take 1 ounce of aloe vera juice on an empty stomach upon rising. Also, make fresh cabbage juice, adding an apple to make it more palatable if necessary. A medical study showed that drinking cabbage juice regularly heals ulcerations.

The amino acid L-glutamine works by nourishing the cells that line the stomach so they can repair themselves. It also contains cancer-preventing agents called glucosinolates. Follow package instructions for taking L-glutamine, or glutamine as it is also known, or take 6 milligrams daily.

Stomach Cancer   Along with the approach outlined under "Cancer" on page 170, follow this additional information specific to stomach cancer.

Consume large amounts of chlorophyll—the green color in plants. Dr. Otto Warburg, 1931 winner of the Nobel Prize for Physiology and Medicine, discovered that oxygen deprivation at the cellular level is a major cause of cancer. Chlorophyll increases cellular oxygenation. While wheatgrass juice is the richest source of chlorophyll, other green vegetables are excellent sources of dietary chlorophyll. Try making green drinks from the juice of fresh green vegetables like kale, collards, spinach, celery, and cucumber. (You can add a small amount of fresh carrot or apple juice for palatability.) I recommend drinking 8 cups of fresh vegetable juice daily for as long as you have stomach cancer. Dilute the juice at a ratio of 50:50 with pure water.

You can also take chlorophyll supplements such as spirulina, chlorella, barley juice powder, alfalfa, or many of the green-food powders available in health food stores. Simply add 1 teaspoon to a glass of juice or a blended drink.

Ulcers Ulcers are lesions in the digestive tract that are usually linked to the bacteria *Helicobacter pylori*. If you have ulcers, you must avoid smoking and coffee. Do not take aspirin, ibuprofen, or other anti-inflammatory drugs, which can aggravate ulcers.

If you suffer from ulcers, there are many things you can do to help ease your symptoms. Eat a high-fiber diet with plenty of whole grains, legumes, and fresh fruits and vegetables. Aloe vera juice is a proven therapy to heal inflamed stomach and intestinal walls and ulcers, so take 1 ounce in the morning on an empty stomach. Also, as a medical study showed that drinking cabbage juice regularly helps to heal ulcerations, try making fresh cabbage juice, with an apple added to make it more palatable (dilute the juice at a 50:50 ratio with pure water).

Studies show that licorice root accelerates the healing of ulcers. Use deglycyrrhizinated licorice (DGL), which is effective but does not upset the body's sodium-potassium balance, and follow package instructions. Ulcer sufferers may also benefit from a green food supplement such as spirulina, chlorella, barley juice powder, or alfalfa, available in health food stores. Simply add 1 teaspoon to a glass of juice or a blended drink.

Other herbs that promote healing of ulcers include meadowsweet, marshmallow root, slippery elm, and mallow. Avoid meadowsweet if you are allergic to aspirin, since it contains aspirin's active ingredient, salicylic acid. Calendula is an herb that helps if the ulcers are bleeding. Drink 3 cups of tea made from steeping 1 to 2 teaspoons of the dried herb (any single herb or combination of those mentioned above) in 1 cup of boiling water for 10 minutes.

Supplementing with the amino acid L-glutamine works by nourishing the cells that line the stomach and esophagus so they can repair themselves. Take 6 milligrams daily with meals or follow the instructions on the package.

Ear Infections and Earaches

There are different types of ear infections, but outer and middle ear infections are the most common. Swimmer's ear is an outer ear infection, while most childhood ear infections occur in the middle ear. In young children, the eustachian tubes (which protect, aerate, and drain the middle ear) are not fully formed and as a result are vulnerable breeding areas for bacteria that can cause ear infections. The eardrums can even rupture due to middle ear infections.

Unfortunately, the most common treatment for ear infections and earaches is antibiotics. Yet research shows that antibiotics are ineffective for most childhood ear infections.[10] That's why I recommend the Phytozyme Cure for ear infections as a natural nonpharmaceutical remedy to this painful condition.

The Phytozyme Cure for Ear Infections
The Diet
Most people suffering from ear infections or earaches are eating more protein foods, namely meat, than their body can handle. To address these concerns, follow the Phytozyme Cure Protein Type diet in Chapter 4.

Emphasize foods that contain alpha-carotene, anthocyanins, beta-carotene, curcumin, hesperetin, resveratrol, and tannins in your diet. See the chart "Phytonutrients: What They Do and Where to Find

Them" on page 32 for more about these specific phytonutrients. Also, eat lots of fresh garlic—it contains natural antibacterial and antiviral substances.

If you suffer from ear infections or earaches, completely eliminate dairy from your diet. Dairy is mucous-forming, and earaches and ear infections may actually be symptoms of a dairy allergy. The same is true for children: most ear infections improve dramatically when children eat a dairy-free diet. Also, be sure to eliminate sugar until the ear infection or earache is gone, and follow a low-sugar diet afterward.

Supplementing the Diet

Supplementing your diet with a high-quality full-spectrum digestive enzyme formula that includes amylase, lipase, and protease, among other enzymes, is also beneficial. Take 1 to 3 enzyme capsules or tablets with every meal to help your body break down the carbohydrates, fats, and proteins in your food into the natural sugars, essential fatty acids, and amino acids needed for optimal healing.

It can also be helpful to supplement with one or more of the following enzymes between meals on an empty stomach: bromelain, chymotrypsin, mucolase, papain, protease, serrapeptidase, superoxide dismutase (SOD), or trypsin, or try a single product that includes some or all of these enzymes. Start by taking 1 capsule or tablet of your chosen enzyme(s) on an empty stomach 20 minutes before or at least 1 hour after meals, three times daily. You can gradually increase that amount to 3 capsules or tablets at a time, three times daily, or more with the guidance of a nutritional medicine practitioner who is experienced in systemic enzyme therapy.

High doses of vitamin C can be helpful to treating ear infections by acting as an antihistamine and assisting with lessening inflammation. Adults should take 2000 milligrams three times daily; children can take 500 milligrams per year of age in doses of 500 milligrams at a time. (For example, a two year old could take 500 milligrams at a time, up to a dose of 1000 milligrams a day). For children 13 years of age and older, the adult dosage is appropriate.

Zinc is a helpful mineral to boost immunity and ward off infections, and I recommend taking 50 milligrams daily to treat earaches and infections.

Echinacea can be helpful to reduce the amount of healing time and to ward off future infections. Usually echinacea is taken as a tincture (alcohol or glycerin; children should take glycerin-based rather than alcohol-based), so simply follow the dosage instructions on the package. Also, I recommend taking 2 capsules of probiotics nightly at bedtime on an empty stomach, since they have been proven helpful for ear infections.

Another excellent option for treating ear infections in adults and children is ear oil. You can purchase Saint-John's-wort oil for this purpose in most health food stores. Or, you can gently warm several cloves of fresh garlic in olive oil in a small saucepan, then remove the garlic and pour the oil into a sterilized bottle. (Don't use the oil when it is hot—wait for it to cool first.) Place a drop or two of the oil in each ear several times daily. Massage another drop or two into the external part of the ear, jaw, and below the ear several times daily.

Fibromyalgia

Fibromyalgia syndrome is a complex pain disorder characterized by generalized fatigue, chronic headaches, sleep disturbances, neurological and psychological complaints, joint swelling, numbness or tingling sensations, irritable bowel syndrome, stress, menstrual cramps in women, restless legs, irritable bladder, poor memory, and temporomandibular joint (TMJ) syndrome.

While people tend to self-diagnose, fibromyalgia is a serious disorder that should be diagnosed only by a physician. To arrive at a medical diagnosis, a physician will examine you for several basic criteria that are implicated in the syndrome:

- widespread pain in all four quadrants of the body for at least three months in a row;

- tenderness in at least 11 of the 18 tender points linked to fibro-myalgia; and
- generalized achiness or stiffness of at least three sites on the body for at least three months in a row.

The physician will also order medical tests to rule out disorders with similar symptoms.

Like other conditions classified as a syndrome, fibromyalgia is a collection of seemingly unconnected symptoms with no apparent cause. While there are many symptoms, the main one in fibromyalgia is unaccountable pain ("myo" means muscle, "algia" means pain) in the muscles. It is actually a form of arthritis that may have a hormonal component—it affects women to men in a ratio of seven to one. The cause of this painful syndrome is uncertain, but it often starts after an illness, injury, or forceful trauma such as a motor vehicle accident. Many researchers believe these factors may damage the central nervous system, causing severe bodily pain.

In controlled clinical studies, none of the major classes of medications commonly prescribed for fibromyalgia (antidepressants, sleep aids, anxiolytics, sedatives, muscle relaxants, and nonsteroidal anti-inflammatory drugs or NSAIDs) had any significant benefit to people suffering from this syndrome.

Using a natural, holistic, and comprehensive approach that targets the main areas affected by the syndrome, many people experience symptom reversal or a complete recovery.

The Phytozyme Cure for Fibromyalgia
The Diet
People suffering from fibromyalgia can be deficient in any or all of the enzymes needed to digest carbohydrates, fats, or proteins. If, after taking the quizzes in Chapter 4, you found that you were a Phytozyme Cure Carb, Fat, or Protein Type, follow the diet for that particular type. If you could not determine one clear type, follow the Phytozyme Cure Combination Type diet.

Emphasize foods that contain alpha-carotene, anthocyanin, astaxanthin, beta-carotene, capsaicin, catechins, curcumin, ellagic acid, ferulic acid, hesperetin, lipoic acid, proanthocyanidin, silymarin, tannins, and terpene limonoids in your diet. See the chart "Phytonutrients: What They Do and Where to Find Them" on page 32 for more about these specific phytonutrients.

Allergies appear to play a role in fibromyalgia. The most common ones of fibromyalgia sufferers are wheat, gluten, milk and dairy products, sugar and artificial sweeteners, alcoholic beverages, caffeine, and food additives like artificial color. Most of these foods and additives cause or aggravate inflammation in the body.

In a study presented at the American Association for the Advancement of Science, fibromyalgia sufferers were given blood tests to determine possible allergies to 340 foods, food additives, environmental chemicals, and medications. After four months of eliminating those allergens, most people showed significant improvement. They continued to improve after six months and experienced a 50 percent reduction in pain, a 40 percent reduction in depression symptoms, 30 percent less stiffness, and 50 percent more energy.

If you suffer from fibromyalgia, eat a diet high in *raw* fruits and vegetables (emphasize the vegetables). Simply add a large raw salad to your lunch and dinner, have fruit at breakfast, and snack on vegetable crudités and raw nuts and seeds. (My book *The Life Force Diet* tells you more about following a raw food diet and includes delicious raw food recipes.)

Drink 8 to 10 cups of pure water every day (limiting the quantity with meals to 1/2 cup to take nutritional supplements) or freshly made vegetable juices, diluted with water to a 50:50 ratio.

Supplementing the Diet

Supplementing your diet with a high-quality full-spectrum digestive enzyme formula that includes amylase, lipase, and protease, among other enzymes, is also beneficial to easing the pain from fibromyalgia. Take 1 to 3 enzyme capsules or tablets with every meal to help your body break down the carbohydrates, fats, and proteins in your food into the natural sugars, essential fatty acids, and amino acids needed for optimal healing.

It can also be helpful to supplement with one or more of the following enzymes between meals on an empty stomach: protease, serrapeptidase, superoxide dismutase (SOD), or trypsin, or try a single product that includes some or all of these enzymes. Start with 1 capsule or tablet of your chosen enzyme(s) on an empty stomach 20 minutes before or at least 1 hour after meals, three times daily. You can gradually increase that amount to 3 capsules or tablets at a time, three times daily, or more with the guidance of a nutritional medicine practitioner who is experienced in systemic enzyme therapy.

Proteolytic (protein-digesting) enzymes are highly effective in healing the soft tissue damage and resulting pain linked to fibromyalgia. While a high-quality full-spectrum enzyme supplement is recommended along with every meal to support digestion and nutrient absorption, proteolytic enzymes should also be taken on an empty stomach to reduce inflammation and pain because, just like our bodies, they are made up of protein substances. These enzymes also aid in the healing of injured tissue.

Bromelain, which is found in pineapples, is one of the best proteolytic enzymes for fibromyalgia. While eating pineapple is moderation is good for fibromyalgia symptoms, it is essential to take bromelain as a supplement between meals for the most potent anti-inflammatory and anti-pain properties. Remember: Foods contain only enough enzymes to digest the food, not to work on inflammatory substances and toxins within the tissues. Take 3 to 5 capsules of a 5000 mcu (milk clotting unit) potency of bromelain twice daily.

Supplement with curcumin and ginger for pain. Use 1 to 5 grams of gingerroot daily to increase circulation to the muscles and to reduce pain.

Coenzyme Q10 (CoQ10) is also beneficial for energy production to enable muscle healing and to combat fatigue associated with fibromyalgia. By taking CoQ10 with the herb ginkgo biloba, you can increase energy levels, improve memory, and increase oxygen and energy to muscles for tissue healing. I recommend that you take 200 milligrams of CoQ10 and 200 milligrams of ginkgo biloba daily.

Magnesium is one of the most critical minerals for fibromyalgia sufferers. It is required for your body to produce a substance called adenosine triphosphate (ATP), which you need for energy. Magnesium is found in dark green leafy vegetables, legumes, nuts, and seeds, which you should introduce into your diet. As for supplements, while the dose varies for each individual, approximately 1500 milligrams per day is ideal. And when you're at the health food store looking at available products, notice that some magnesium supplements are accompanied by malic acid, which is an important compound for treating fibromyalgia. I recommend 1200 to 2400 milligrams of malic acid daily to combat pain.

As for herbs, kava (*Piper methysticum*) is an analgesic herb whose potency ranks between aspirin and morphine, making it an excellent choice for most pain disorders, including fibromyalgia. It is also a muscle relaxant and sleep aid, making it particularly suitable for this condition. Unlike tranquilizers, kava does not create negative morning symptoms in those taking this herb. Because it has been linked to liver damage, however, it should be used only under the guidance of a health care practitioner.

Other anti-pain foods and herbs are willow bark, boswellia serrata (Indian frankincense), and guggul gum. Willow bark is a good herb choice, since it works primarily on the joints. Take 500 milligrams three times daily. However, you should avoid willow bark if you are allergic to salicylic acid or aspirin.

Also, I recommend taking 2 probiotic capsules nightly at bedtime on an empty stomach to counter bacterial imbalances linked to fibromyalgia.

Some researchers indicate that fibromyalgia sufferers appear to have lower than normal levels of a liver hormone called somatomedin C, which aids tissue repair during the deepest phase of sleep. But because many sufferers have trouble sleeping, their bodies do not secrete enough of this hormone. Drinking herbal teas in the evening, made of valerian or passionflower, can help with sleep quality.

Finally, I do understand that the pain and fatigue that many fibromyalgia patients suffer can make beginning an exercise program difficult. But research shows that when sufferers gradually increase their activity levels, their symptoms improve. In a small Swedish study of the effect of pool exercise on fibromyalgia suffers, researchers found lasting improvements in symptom severity and physical and social function. So try to incorporate at least some light physical activity into your day whenever you can.

Headaches and Migraines

There are many types of headaches: tension headaches, sinus headaches, cluster headaches, classic migraines, and common migraines. For simplicity, I have grouped headaches and migraines together, but they are actually very different. Migraines are much more than just bad headaches. As traditional naturopath Linda Page, PhD, describes them in her book *Linda Page's Healthy Healing*, "They're a total body assault." Having suffered with migraines for many years after severe car accident injuries, I can attest to that.

First, let's review the different types of headaches:

- *Tension headaches* are the result of muscle contractions in the temples and/or back of the head, usually as a result of stress or fatigue. They typically last for hours or days and feel like one's head is in the grip of a vise.
- *Sinus headaches* result from inflammation and congestion in the sinuses. They usually involve a dull ache over the eyes, as well as sleeplessness and irritability.
- *Cluster headaches* are severe headaches that come on suddenly and frequently—usually two or more extremely severe headaches daily. They are usually accompanied by light sensitivity, movement sensitivity, and nausea. More likely to affect

men, they appear to be connected to testosterone imbalances, repressed anger, and histamine reactions (allergic reactions). They are called cluster headaches because they cluster over the forehead and eyes and can even cause distorted vision.

- *Classic migraines* are caused by the constriction and dilation of blood vessels in the brain, scalp, and face. They involve severe throbbing or stabbing pain that is preceded by seeing an aura and having a sudden sensitivity to light and odors, as well as nausea, vomiting, visual disturbances, chills, and fevers. They usually last up to three or four days.

- *Common migraines* are similar to classic migraines, except the sufferer does not see the aura before a migraine's onset. They come with the same severe pain and visual disturbances, distortion of smells and tastes, weakness, and confusion. One of the main causes of migraines is hormonal imbalance, particularly that of estrogen and testosterone.

Headaches can result from emotional stresses; food allergies; eyestrain from excessive computer work or television viewing; pinched nerves (particularly in the neck); constipation; excess caffeine, salt, or sugar; consumption of the neurotoxins MSG or aspartame; low blood sugar levels; PMS; a sluggish liver; herpes simplex infection; *Candida albicans* overgrowth; heavy metal poisoning, and the use of certain drugs like Viagra, or overuse of nonsteroidal anti-inflammatory drugs (NSAIDs) like aspirin and ibuprofen.

The Phytozyme Cure for Headaches and Migraines
The Diet
People suffering from headaches can be deficient in any or all of the enzymes needed to digest carbohydrates, fats, or proteins. If, after taking the quizzes in Chapter 4, you found that you were a Phytozyme Cure Carb, Fat, or Protein Type, follow the diet for that particular type. If you could not determine one clear type, follow the Phytozyme Cure Combination Type diet.

It is imperative to get the junk out of your diet (I tell you how in Chapter 3), as many of these substances cause headaches in people who are vulnerable to them. If you get headaches or migraine, avoid excess sugar, artificial sweeteners like aspartame and Splenda, artificial colors and flavors, preservatives, trans fats, and MSG.

Emphasize foods that contain alpha carotene, anthocyanins, astaxanthin, beta-carotene, capsaicin, catechins, curcumin, ellagic acid, ferulic acid, hesperetin, lipoic acid, proanthocyanidin, silymarin, and terpene limonoids in your diet. See the chart "Phytonutrients: What They Do and Where to Find Them" on page 32 for more about these specific phytonutrients.

Supplementing the Diet

Supplementing your diet with a high-quality full-spectrum digestive enzyme formula that includes amylase, lipase, and protease, among other enzymes, is also beneficial. Take 1 to 3 enzyme capsules or tablets with every meal to help your body break down the carbohydrates, fats, and proteins in your food into the natural sugars, essential fatty acids, and amino acids needed for optimal healing.

It can also be helpful to supplement with one or more of the following enzymes between meals on an empty stomach: bromelain, mucolase (specifically for sinus headaches), superoxide dismutase (SOD), or trypsin, or a single product that includes some or all of these enzymes. Start with 1 capsule or tablet of your chosen enzyme(s) on an empty stomach 20 minutes before or at least 1 hour after meals, three times daily. You can gradually increase that amount to 3 capsules or tablets at a time, three times daily, or more with the guidance of a nutritional medicine practitioner who is experienced in systemic enzyme therapy.

The B-complex vitamins are integral to many functions in the body, including the management of headaches. Take a 100-milligram B-complex vitamin. If you are suffering from either type of migraines, take an additional 400 milligrams of niacin (vitamin B3) daily. It may be necessary to take niacin in divided doses to avoid the harmless but sometimes uncomfortable symptom called niacin flushing. Avoid extra niacin if you suffer from cluster headaches.

Magnesium is nature's relaxation nutrient, and it is extremely valuable in the treatment of headaches of all kinds. Take 800 milligrams daily to help relax muscles and improve neurotransmitter function in the brain. The nutrient 5-HTP is also proven to help calm stress reactions, and you may benefit from a daily dose of 50 milligrams.

Be sure you're getting adequate fatty acids by taking 1 to 2 grams of fish oil capsules or flaxseed oil capsules daily. Fish oils have anti-pain and anti-inflammatory properties helpful for headaches.

If you are a woman who suffers from hormone-related migraines that occur during your periods, take the herb dong quai throughout the month but especially the week before your period.

If you began experiencing headaches or migraines following neck injuries, you may find massage therapy, chiropractic treatment, acupuncture, or acupressure helpful. I found massage therapy, along with the healthy diet I have outlined in *The Phytozyme Cure,* to be extremely helpful in dealing with my own migraines that developed after a severe car accident.

Also, you may find meditation, stress reduction techniques, and deep breathing exercises beneficial. Many headaches improve dramatically from increased oxygen through deep breathing or through oxygen inhalation therapy.

Heart Disease

Also known as cardiovascular disease, heart disease is a collection of disorders affecting the heart and blood vessels. Heart disease is the number one killer in the United States and Canada. That's truly sad when you consider that most heart disease is completely preventable.

Cholesterol levels were once believed to be one of the greatest determinants of heart disease risk. However, most physicians now recognize that homocysteine levels provide a much greater understanding of one's risk for heart disease. Let's look at homocysteine and how it is linked to heart disease.

Homocysteine is a type of protein that is produced by the body and exists in the blood. It is ideally found in low levels. The body normally turns homocysteine into beneficial substances such as glutathione or S-adenosylmethionine (SAMe).

High levels of homocysteine damage arteries, the brain, and genetic material (DNA) and can increase the risk for over 50 diseases, including Alzheimer's disease, cancer, depression, diabetes, heart attack, stroke, and rheumatoid arthritis.[11]

Risk Factors for Heart Disease

Numerous risk factors can increase your chances of having high levels of homocysteine in your body:[12]

- Genetics (a family history of heart disease, strokes, cancer, Alzheimer's disease, schizophrenia, or diabetes, or the MTHFR enzyme gene mutation)
- Folate deficiency (less than 900 micrograms/day)
- Increased age
- Gender (males are more at risk)
- Estrogen deficiency
- Excessive alcohol, coffee, or tea intake
- Smoking
- Sedentary lifestyle
- Hostility and repressed anger
- Inflammatory bowel disease like celiac, Crohn's, or ulcerative colitis
- Helicobacter pylori–generated ulcers
- Pregnancy
- Poor diet that's high in fat, dairy, and salt

A buildup of homocysteine in the blood is called hyperhomocysteinemia, which is linked to increased formation of plaque on blood vessel walls and clogging and hardening of the arteries—atherosclerosis.

Researchers at the Department of Cardiology at Southampton General Hospital in England reviewed 92 studies on homocysteine. According to their findings, every five-unit (millimole/liter) increase in homocysteine measured in the blood increased the risk for heart disease by 42 percent in people with the MTHFR gene mutation and by 32 percent in those without the gene mutation. The risk for stroke went up by 65 percent in those with the genetic mutation and by 59 percent in those without the mutation. The researchers concluded that there is "strong evidence that the association between homocysteine and cardiovascular disease is causal," meaning that high homocysteine levels cause heart disease.[13]

Homocysteine and Other Health Conditions

Breast and colon cancer, as well as leukemia and other cancers, have been linked to high homocysteine levels.[14] Damage to DNA is a cancer trigger, and high homocysteine levels make your DNA more vulnerable to damage and difficult for your body to repair once the damage is done. According to Patrick Holford, founder of the Institute for Optimum Nutrition, if you lower your homocysteine levels, you can cut your cancer risk by more than half.[15]

It is also possible that homocysteine plays a role in diabetes. Research has found that the abnormally raised insulin levels found in most diabetics disrupt the body's ability to lower and maintain healthy levels of homocysteine.[16]

In addition, homocysteine is strongly linked to brain damage and the risk of Alzheimer's disease. According to research, lower levels of homocysteine dramatically reduce the risk of Alzheimer's disease.[17]

But we are still not sure exactly how far-reaching the damage caused by high homocysteine levels can be. Research published in the *American Journal of Clinical Nutrition* found that there was a strong correlation between homocysteine and "all causes of mortality."[18]

The Phytozyme Cure for Heart Disease
The Diet

Most people suffering from heart disease are eating more fat or protein than their body can handle. To address these concerns, follow the Phytozyme Cure Protein Type, outlined in Chapter 4, if you have heart disease combined with high blood pressure or hypertension, or the Phytozyme Cure Fat Type diet.

Lowering Homocysteine Levels with a Healthy Diet

You can reduce homocysteine levels in your body by following these simple suggestions:[19]

- Eat less fatty meat and more fish and vegetable protein.
- Eat green vegetables and leafy greens, which are high in B-complex vitamins, including vitamin B6, B12, and folate.
- Eat whole grains, which are high in B-complex vitamins.
- Eat a clove of garlic a day.
- Reduce your salt intake.
- Cut back on tea and coffee.
- Limit your alcohol.
- Reduce your stress.
- Stop smoking.
- Correct an estrogen deficiency if you have one (there are many natural ways to do so without resorting to estrogen replacement therapy).
- Supplement with a multivitamin every day.
- Take homocysteine-reducing nutrient supplements. (I tell you about these a bit later in this section—see the "Homocysteine-Reducing Nutrients" box.)

Emphasize foods that contain anthocyanin, astaxanthin, beta-sitosterol, catechins, chlorogenic acid, curcumin, hesperetin, lipoic acid, lutein, lycopene, naringin, pectin, proanthocyanidin, and resveratrol in your diet. See the chart "Phytonutrients: What They Do and Where to Find Them" on page 32 for more about these specific phytonutrients.

Supplementing the Diet

Supplementing your diet with a high-quality full-spectrum digestive enzyme formula that includes amylase, lipase, and protease, among other enzymes, is also beneficial. Take 1 to 3 enzyme capsules or tablets with every meal to help your body break down the carbohydrates, fats, and proteins in your food into the natural sugars, essential fatty acids, and amino acids needed for optimal healing.

It can also be helpful to supplement with one or more of the following enzymes between meals on an empty stomach: bromelain, catalase, lipase, nattokinase, protease, serrapeptidase, superoxide dismutase (SOD), or trypsin, or a single product that includes some or all of these enzymes. Start with 1 capsule or tablet of your chosen enzyme(s) on an empty stomach 20 minutes before or at least 1 hour after meals, three times daily. You can gradually increase that amount to 3 capsules or tablets at a time, three times daily, or more with the guidance of a nutritional medicine practitioner who is experienced in systemic enzyme therapy.

Homocysteine-Reducing Nutrients

There are many nutrients required to lower homocysteine levels in the body. A deficiency in even a single one can impair the body's ability to neutralize the harmful homocysteine, resulting in higher risk of serious illness. In addition to some dietary and lifestyle changes, taking a few important supplements can spell the difference between health and illness.

Supplementing with B-complex vitamins can be helpful, since they are required to activate the enzymes that turn homocysteine into glutathione or SAMe. Without adequate amounts of these vitamins, homocysteine will not be converted to these beneficial substances, resulting in dangerously high levels of homocysteine and potentially low levels of beneficial glutathione and SAMe. Research shows that supplementing with folate and vitamin B12 can make the deficient enzyme work more effectively. In addition to adequate B12 and folate, your body needs adequate levels of vitamins B2, B6, zinc, and trimethylglycine (TMG) to metabolize homocysteine.[20] All of these B-vitamins can be found in a single B-complex supplement, so take a 100-milligram B-complex vitamin daily.

In a study published in the journal *Clinical Therapy*, researchers found that supplementing with a multivitamin containing vitamins B6, B12, and folate for 26 weeks decreased homocysteine concentrations. In another study published in the journal *Stroke*, stroke victims who supplemented with vitamins B6, B12, and folate for one year experienced a 24 percent drop in homocysteine levels compared to the placebo group, whose homocysteine levels rose slightly.[21]

Irritable Bowel Syndrome

Irritable bowel syndrome (IBS) is a common condition involving alternating diarrhea and constipation, abdominal pain, bloating, mucous in stools, and irregular bowel movements. It is usually diagnosed by ruling out other intestinal diagnoses. IBS typically comes and goes over the years. To help manage the symptoms, follow the dietary and supplement suggestions under "Colitis and Crohn's Disease" on page 179 and "Digestive Disorders" on page 189.

Lupus

The full name for lupus is systemic lupus erythematosus. It is an autoimmune viral inflammatory disease that is estimated to affect close to 2 million Americans. The immune system attacks its own connective tissue and joints, resulting in arthritis-type symptoms. The lymph nodes and kidneys can also become inflamed. In severe cases, the heart, brain, and nervous system can degenerate.

There are many symptoms of lupus, including severe fatigue; depression; rough skin patches; chronic nail fungus; sensitivity to light; dry eyes; migraines; anemia; arthritic-feeling joints; inflammation around the mouth, cheeks, and nose; low-grade fevers, and memory lapses and forgetfulness.

A study in the *New England Journal of Medicine* indicates that up to 10 percent of lupus cases may actually be caused by drug reactions.[22] Some health experts believe that lupus may be caused by food sensitivities, severe stress, diabetic tendencies, *Candida albicans,* or a chronic viral infection linked to having taken excessive amounts of antibiotics or other prescription drugs.

The Phytozyme Cure for Lupus
The Diet

People suffering from lupus can be deficient in any or all of the enzymes needed to digest carbohydrates, fats, or proteins. If, after taking the quizzes in Chapter 4, you found that you were a Phytozyme Cure Carb, Fat, or Protein Type, follow the diet for that particular type. If you could not determine one clear type, follow the Phytozyme Cure Combination Type diet.

To get the best results from a lupus-specific diet, emphasize foods that contain alpha carotene, capsaicin, curcumin, ellagic acid, hesperetin, lipoic acid, lycopene, proanthocyanidin, resveratrol, silymarin, sulforaphane, tangeretin, and terpene limonoids in your diet. See the chart "Phytonutrients: What They Do and Where to Find Them" on page 32 for more about these specific phytonutrients.

Many people with lupus suffer from food sensitivities that aggravate their condition. Some of the main food sensitivities are corn, wheat, gluten, rye bread, pork (including bacon), beef, eggs, coffee, dairy products, chocolate, and oranges. I highly recommend eliminating these foods, as well as alcohol and fried foods, from your diet.

Also, alfalfa seeds have been linked to symptoms of lupus. While most people are not in the habit of eating alfalfa seeds, if you suffer from this particular condition, it might be wise to avoid alfalfa sprouts and green powders containing alfalfa grass.

Adopting an alkalizing diet made up of about 70 percent vegetables and with limited meat and dairy products can substantially help to reduce pain and other symptoms of lupus. (The topic of pH balancing in your body is quite comprehensive and requires a full book to do it justice. If you want to read more about pH balancing, consult my book *The Ultimate pH Solution*.)

Supplementing the Diet

Supplementing your diet with a high-quality full-spectrum digestive enzyme formula that includes amylase, bromelain, cellulose, lipase, papain, protease, serrapeptidase, superoxide dismutase (SOD), and trypsin, among other enzymes, is also beneficial. Take 1 to 3 enzyme capsules or tablets with every meal to help your body break down the carbohydrates, fats, and proteins in your food into the natural sugars, essential fatty acids, and amino acids needed for optimal healing.

It can also be helpful to supplement with one or more of the following enzymes between meals on an empty stomach: bromelain, cellulose, papain, protease, serrapeptidase, superoxide dismutase (SOD), or trypsin, or a single product that includes some or all of these enzymes. Start with 3 capsules or tablets of your chosen enzyme(s) on an empty stomach 20 minutes before or at least 1 hour after meals, three times daily. You can gradually increase that amount to 5 capsules or tablets at a time, three times daily, or more with the guidance of a nutritional medicine practitioner experienced in systemic enzyme therapy.

Alternatively, take 1500 milligrams a day of bromelain in divided doses between meals to reduce inflammation. You may also achieve this effect by taking 1000 milligrams of quercetin a day with meals.

Many other supplements are helpful in easing the symptoms of lupus:

- Vitamin D, 2000 IU daily, to help regulate the immune system.
- Vitamin A, 10,000 IU daily, to support a balanced immune response.
- Vitamin C, 6000 milligrams, in divided doses of 2000 milligrams, to reduce inflammation.
- DHA-EPA from flaxseed oil or fish oil, 1000 to 3000 milligrams of fish or flaxseed oil daily. That's about 500 milligrams of EPA and 360 milligrams of DHA daily if you choose an EPA-DHA–type product.
- Niacinamide, 3000 milligrams daily (alternatively, you can use niacin, but divide the doses, since it can cause flushing).
- Methylsulfonylmethane (MSM) occurs naturally in the body and is found in some foods, particularly green vegetables. Take 5000 milligrams daily to counter pain and inflammation. Because it has blood-thinning properties, avoid using MSM if you are taking pharmaceutical blood thinners.
- Alpha lipoic acid, 300 milligrams daily, as an antioxidant to scavenge free radicals linked to lupus.
- SAMe, 400 to 600 milligrams daily, to help protect joints and balance brain chemicals.
- CoQ10, 300 milligrams daily, to boost cellular energy available for healing.
- Vitamin E, 800 IU daily, may help lower inflammatory compounds in the body.
- Devil's claw is an excellent anti-inflammatory and anti-pain herb. Take it in capsules or as an extract (following instructions for the brand you choose).

- Aloe vera juice, 2 ounces every morning on an empty stomach, to help heal a leaky gut, which is often a problem in autoimmune disorders like lupus.
- The hormone DHEA may also be beneficial; however, it is available only by prescription in Canada. Consult a naturally minded physician.

Because intestinal yeast overgrowth can play a role in lupus, follow the dietary and supplement suggestions for "Yeast Infections" on page 245.

Multiple Sclerosis

Known by most people as "MS," multiple sclerosis is a serious, degenerative disease of the central nervous system. Nerves are delicate structures that have a protective coating called myelin. In multiple sclerosis, the myelin degenerates, leaving parts of the nerves vulnerable, scarred, or damaged. If that happens, the affected nerves begin to malfunction.

MS is the most common neurological affliction, affecting over a quarter million people in the United States. People usually develop MS between the ages of 20 and 40, but the disease can occur at any age. Two-thirds of MS sufferers are women.

The symptoms of the disease depend on which nerves become damaged; however, MS has numerous common symptoms, including exhaustion, dizziness, loss of balance, blurry vision, constipation, tremors, staggering gait, bowel and bladder incontinence, numb or weak limbs, impaired speech, facial paralysis, poor coordination, nausea and vomiting, blindness, and paralysis. One common pattern in people diagnosed with MS is that the symptoms and attacks occur in cycles, known as exacerbations and remissions. Some people even go into lifelong remission.

It is still a mystery why the myelin sheath degenerates in some people but not in others. The medical community has not isolated a single cause of MS, but there are many theories. The most prominent theory is that MS is an autoimmune disorder in which white blood cells think the myelin is a foreign invader and attack it. Another theory is that MS is the result of a virus or other pathogenic invasion, either bacterial or fungal. Other factors that may play a role in MS are chronic stress and/or stress hormone imbalances, immunizations, free radical damage, environmental toxins and heavy-metal toxicity, poor nutrition (particularly a vitamin D deficiency), and food allergies.

Multiple sclerosis has become increasingly common in Canada and the United States, but it is still rare in tropical, eastern, and developing countries. Some research links the frequency of MS to higher geographical latitudes, making Canada, the northern United States, England, Scandinavia, and other northern European countries especially vulnerable to increased incidence. Researchers are uncertain as to why this might be the case, but some studies link higher sun exposure between the ages of 6 and 15 to a reduced risk of MS, and believe that vitamin D from sun exposure helps prevent the disease.

It is also well documented that extreme, chronic stress and poor nutrition can worsen MS, and some experts believe that these factors may also contribute to the disease's onset. Many environmental toxins can create symptoms similar to MS and can even damage the myelin or the body's own DNA. Food sensitivities appear to play a role in worsening MS symptoms. We often incorrectly assume that food sensitivities manifest as anaphylactic shock (as in the case of a peanut allergy) or in hay fever–type symptoms. But they are more typically implicated in autoimmune disorders and chronic inflammatory conditions in the body.

The Phytozyme Cure for Multiple Sclerosis
The Diet

People suffering from MS can be deficient in any or all of the enzymes needed to digest carbohydrates, fats, or proteins. If, after taking the quizzes in Chapter 4, you found that you were a Phytozyme Cure Carb, Fat, or Protein Type, follow the diet for that particular type. If you could not determine one clear type, follow The Phytozyme Cure Combination Type diet.

Emphasize foods that contain alpha carotene, capsaicin, curcumin, ellagic acid, hesperetin, lipoic acid, lycopene, proanthocyanidin, resveratrol, silymarin, sulforaphane, tangeretin, and terpene limonoids in your diet. See the chart "Phytonutrients: What They Do and Where to Find Them" on page 32 for more about these specific phytonutrients.

Dairy and wheat allergies often manifest in autoimmune disorders, causing the body to attack healthy nerves or tissues. Eliminate *all* dairy and wheat products from your diet. That includes milk, butter, cream, ice cream, cheese (including soy, rice, and almond cheeses made with casein), and whey powder. Pay particular attention to wheat, as it is commonplace in pasta, buns, breads, baked goods, spice mixtures, coatings on chicken or other meat, and soups, and many other foods.

Because free radical damage may play a role in multiple sclerosis, it is important to eat a diet that will not aggravate inflammation and is devoid of harmful substances that increase free radicals in the body. Eliminating free radicals in your system is an important part of *The Phytozyme Cure*, as you know from previous chapters.

Supplementing the Diet

Supplementing your diet with a high-quality full-spectrum digestive enzyme formula that includes amylase, lipase, and protease, among other enzymes, is also beneficial. Take 1 to 3 enzyme capsules or tablets with every meal to help your body break down the carbohydrates, fats, and proteins in your food into the natural sugars, essential fatty acids, and amino acids needed for optimal healing.

It can also be helpful to supplement with one or more of the following enzymes between meals on an empty stomach: bromelain, lipase, papain, protease, serrapeptidase, superoxide dismutase (SOD), or trypsin, or a single product that includes some or all of these enzymes. Start with 3 capsules or tablets of your chosen enzyme(s) on an empty stomach 20 minutes before or at least 1 hour after meals, three times daily. You can gradually increase that amount with the guidance of a nutritional medicine practitioner who is experienced in systemic enzyme therapy.

A full-spectrum digestive enzyme supplement is helpful to lessen food allergy reactions, which in turn lessens the likelihood of other autoimmune reactions. Take 1 to 2 capsules or tablets of a full-spectrum enzyme formulation, containing amylase, lactase, lipase, protease, and other enzymes, with each meal. Take additional enzymes between meals on an empty stomach to lessen inflammation. When the enzymes, particularly protease, have no food to digest, they help break down the by-products of inflammation, which are made up, in part, of protein. The enzymes also can help the body destroy pathogens like bacteria, viruses, and fungi when the enzymes are taken on an empty stomach.

Poor nutrition, particularly vitamin D and/or essential fatty acid deficiency, is often implicated in MS. Daily responsible sun exposure helps the body manufacture vitamin D and is far superior to supplementing this vitamin. Sunscreens block the skin's capacity for this biochemical process. Just 15 minutes of sunlight daily is helpful, even in the winter months. However, it is valuable to supplement with 2000 to 4000 IU of vitamin D daily as well.

Research by Dr. Roy Swank, a professor of neurology at the University of Oregon's medical school, has shown that a diet low in saturated fats with the addition of 1 teaspoon of cod liver oil daily, over long periods of time, can halt the progression of MS.[23] One of Swank's studies was conducted over 34 years. His research and its extensive duration offer promise for people suffering from this troubling disease. As early as 1948, Dr. Swank began treating patients with his diet low in saturated fat. Since that time, other naturally minded physicians have modified his approach by adding flaxseed oil.

Fish oil in high doses, usually between 5 and 20 grams daily, is best for MS. Be sure the source is pure (devoid of heavy metals) and contains both DHA and EPA essential fats. Take your digestive enzyme alongside meals that contain fish or fish oil supplements to assist with digestion and absorption.

In addition to fish oil, take a GLA supplement. "GLA" stands for gamma-linoleic acid, which is usually found in evening primrose and borage oil. GLA is an excellent natural anti-inflammatory remedy.

Probiotics, like those mentioned in Chapter 3, are imperative to a healthy immune system and digestive tract, and help to lessen inflammation and autoimmune reactions. Take 2 capsules nightly on an empty stomach before bed.

To prevent any other nutritional deficiencies, take a high-quality multivitamin and mineral daily with meals.

Vitamin B12 is involved in the formation of healthy myelin to protect the nerves. Take a sublingual (under the tongue) form at a dose between 400 and 800 micrograms daily. Usually sublingual vitamin B12 comes in liquid form or small dissolvable tablets.

Vitamin E is a potent antioxidant and helps to prevent free radical formation in the body. Take 400 IU of mixed tocopherols daily.

Ginkgo biloba is another powerful antioxidant that helps protect the nerves from free radical damage. Take between 60 and 120 milligrams twice daily of a product containing 24 percent glycosides and 6 percent terpene lactones for maximum benefit.

Plant sterols, which are natural plant hormones, are helpful to restore balance to the immune system. Take 20 milligrams three times a day on an empty stomach to help lessen autoimmune reactions.

Osteoporosis

Osteoporosis is a condition that is characterized by low bone mass or loss of bone mass over time. Bones lose their minerals, become porous, and are vulnerable to fractures or breaks. According to some estimates, in the United States there are 10 million people, mostly women, suffering from osteoporosis.

While most physicians cite insufficient calcium as the cause of this condition, there is research that indicates that those nations with the highest calcium intake have the highest rates of osteoporosis. I do believe calcium plays a role, but I also think there are other factors at work, including eating too many acid-forming foods (like sugar) and a vitamin D deficiency, among others. But before we get into the nutrition and supplementation aspects, let's take a minute to consider our bones. They give our bodies structure and play an important role in maintaining our posture, balance, and immune system. But unfortunately, we don't give our bones much thought until they fracture or break. While we often think of them as unchanging concrete-like structures that do not interact much with the rest of our bodies, this idea is not true. Bones are alive—like other tissues in our body. They are made up of living cells and are approximately 50 percent water.

Our bones provide a constant supply of healthy blood to our organs and tissues. They act as mineral bank accounts for our bodies, storing excess minerals until they can be used by the body or excreted. Bones even assist with hormonal balance. They receive chemical messages of what our hormonal systems need from them and then release minerals to assist as necessary.

Thanks to dairy advertising boards, we tend to think of bones as almost exclusively made up of calcium. That belief is inaccurate. Bones are made up of more than two dozen elements, including phosphorus and magnesium. And, of course, calcium. Bones are constantly being rebuilt by cells called osteoblasts and broken down by osteoclasts. Bone becomes weak when the destruction of bones exceeds the rate of rebuilding. To use the bank account analogy again, when we are always withdrawing minerals from our bones but not depositing new minerals, we deplete our bones' supply.

If you always borrowed money from the bank and never repaid it, you would develop credit problems. Eventually, the bank would stop lending to you. When the bones become chronically depleted of minerals they become fragile and weak, vulnerable to various types of illness and injuries. Fractures of the hip are most commonly caused from weakened, demineralized bones.

Osteoporosis affects one out of every four postmenopausal women in the United States.[24] As I noted, the major risk factor for this illness is a chronic insufficiency of calcium, but there are also other important deficiencies related to this condition. So for the Phytozyme Cure, we're going to look at how you can get more calcium, as well as other nutrients, in your diet to prevent osteoporosis and lessen its symptoms.[25]

The Phytozyme Cure for Osteoporosis
The Diet

Most people suffering from osteoporosis are eating more carbohydrates (usually in the form of sugar and sugary foods) and protein (usually in the form of excess meat) than their body can handle, or are suffering from a sugar intolerance. To address these concerns, follow the Phytozyme Cure Carb Type or the Phytozyme Cure Protein Type diet, depending on your quiz results from Chapter 4.

Regardless which of the Phytozyme Cure Type diets you follow, emphasize foods that contain hesperetin, lycopene, and isoflavones (particularly if you are a woman who is menopausal or postmenopausal) in your diet. See the chart "Phytonutrients: What They Do and Where to Find Them" on page 32 for more about these specific phytonutrients.

While dairy industry advertisements might make you think that strengthening bones is simply a matter of eating more dairy products, that isn't the case. You need to include highly usable sources of calcium in your diet, including carrots and carrot juice (diluted 50:50 with water), kale, dark leafy greens, sesame seeds, tahini (sesame butter), broccoli, almonds, almond butter, kelp, oats, and navy beans. Kelp is an excellent choice, since it also provides many other minerals needed for bone healing.

If you are a woman going through menopause or are postmenopausal, you may need to address possible hormone imbalances to ensure proper bone healing. Balancing hormones in women is also imperative to bone health and healing, since estrogen and testosterone help the body to assimilate calcium and other bone-building minerals.

The mineral boron acts as a mild estrogen replacement therapy in postmenopausal women who are at risk of weakened bones. Yet research shows that the average North American obtains only half the amount of boron necessary to prevent bone demineralization. Boron is found in greatest concentrations in fruit, particularly apples, dates, grapes, peaches, pears, and raisins. It is also found in legumes and nuts, especially almonds and hazelnuts, as well as in honey.

Vitamin K is another important nutrient in maintaining strong bones. It is primarily found in green vegetables, which also happen to be a good source of calcium, so green vegetables are an excellent part of a diet to prevent osteoporosis.

Good Sources of Calcium

Most people tend to think only of dairy products like milk, yogurt, and cheese when they think of calcium. But there are many other excellent sources of calcium, including legumes; whole grains; dark green leafy vegetables such as mustard greens, collard greens, turnip greens, kale, spinach, Swiss chard, and salad greens; figs; apricots; rhubarb; calcium-fortified orange juice and soy milk; sardines and salmon with bones; tofu; and blackstrap molasses.

Supplementing the Diet

Supplementing your diet with a high-quality full-spectrum digestive enzyme formula that includes amylase, lipase, and protease, among other enzymes, is also beneficial. Take 1 to 3 enzyme capsules or tablets with every meal to help your body break down the carbohydrates, fats, and proteins in your food into the natural sugars, essential fatty acids, and amino acids needed for optimal bone healing.

It can also be helpful to supplement with one or more of the following enzymes between meals on an empty stomach: lipase or protease, or a single product that includes both of these enzymes. Lipase carries calcium across the intestinal walls and into the blood so your bones can use it, while protease carries calcium in the blood. Start with

1 capsule or tablet of your chosen enzyme(s) on an empty stomach 20 minutes before or at least 1 hour after meals, three times daily. You can gradually increase that amount to 3 capsules or tablets at a time, three times daily, or more with the guidance of a nutritional medicine practitioner who is experienced in systemic enzyme therapy.

The phytonutrient ipriflavone (7-isopropoxy-isoflavone) can also be helpful with osteoporosis, since it inhibits the loss of bone cells. Working with other nutrients, it increases bone mineral density, stimulates bone cells, and increases calcium absorption.

Menopausal or postmenopausal women need between 1200 and 1500 milligrams of calcium per day.[26] And if osteoporosis is a concern for you, it is important to address any other mineral deficiencies you may have. The following minerals are just as important to bone health. Choose a multimineral supplement that contains all of these minerals:

- Boron, to aid the absorption of calcium
- Magnesium, to help the body to absorb and utilize calcium
- Phosphorus, important in bone mineralization and the synthesis of collagen, a glue-like protein that helps to hold everything together
- Potassium, which enhances calcium absorption
- Silica, required for bone collagen formation and healing bone fractures
- Zinc, necessary for bone growth and development and which works synergistically with calcium

Numerous vitamins are also essential to bone health and healing. I recommend that you supplement with the following vitamins to give back the support that your bones give you every day:

- Vitamin A, to aid bone and teeth formation
- B vitamins (6, 9, and 12), to protect the body from a buildup of homocysteine, a protein by-product that interferes with collagen formation needed for bone development and health

- Vitamin C, essential to produce adequate levels of bone collagen
- Vitamin D3 (cholecalciferol), which draws calcium from the blood into the bones, stimulating the absorption of calcium from supplements and the diet to form stronger bones
- Vitamin K, required for the production of osteocalcin (a bone protein), which provides structure to bone tissue and is critical to repair; without it, bones become fragile and break easily

Without adequate vitamins and minerals like those listed above, the bones simply cannot properly absorb calcium. Fortunately, a high-potency and high-quality vitamin and mineral supplement can usually supply all of these vitamins and minerals.

Glucosamine sulfate, an amino sugar that helps with bone formation, is also important to bone health.

I believe that one of the common causes of osteoporosis is vitamin D deficiency, so let's look a bit more at this nutrient and its role in bone health. Research shows that vitamin D is important not only to your overall health but also in preventing osteoporosis. While some foods, including fish and fortified milk, contain vitamin D, the primary source of this vitamin is the sun—your skin makes vitamin D when you are exposed to sunlight. However, most people simply do not get enough vitamin D from sunshine or in their diets. After being out in the sun, your body takes about 48 hours to absorb vitamin D into the blood. In that time, even the soap you use on your skin in the bath or shower binds to the sunlight-initiated precursors to vitamin D before the vitamin has a chance to be absorbed by the body. And for many people with hypothyroidism, the amount of vitamin D that is absorbed either from sunshine, food, or supplementation is greatly reduced. Most people benefit from additional vitamin D in the cholecalciferol form. From 2000 to 4000 IU daily is a suitable dose to aid bone healing and assist with the absorption of calcium.

And finally, leading an active lifestyle is a great defense against osteoporosis. Of course, if you have a fracture that is healing, you need to rest that area. However, after that, it's important to get bone-building exercise. Research from the International Osteoporosis Foundation shows that physical activity is necessary to build and maintain strong bones. Weight-bearing exercises like running, walking, and rebounding are particularly good, as long as your bones are strong enough and have healed.

Overweight and Obesity

According to recent information from the US National Center for Health Statistics, 30 percent of Americans are obese. That's about 60 million people. An additional third of the US population is overweight. That's a staggering two of every three people! Canada isn't much different—23 percent of adults are obese. Obesity rates are also on the rise in Europe and Asia.

Even the percentage of overweight or obese children has tripled in the last three decades. When you consider that being overweight or obese dramatically increases one's likelihood of experiencing serious illnesses like heart disease and diabetes, this is a serious problem.

But addressing excess weight or obesity doesn't have to be a battle, especially with the Phytozyme Cure on your side. Simply making healthier food choices rich in phytonutrients, eating frequently throughout the day to stabilize blood sugar, supplementing with important enzymes and other supplements, and exercising regularly can cause healthy, long-term weight loss.

The Phytozyme Cure for Overweight and Obesity
The Diet
Most people dealing with excess weight or obesity are eating more carbohydrates or fat than their bodies can handle, or they are experiencing deficiencies in the enzymes to digest these foods. To address these concerns, follow the Phytozyme Cure Carbohydrate Type or the Phytozyme Cure Fat Type diet outlined in Chapter 4.

Emphasize foods that contain anthocyanin, astaxanthin, capsaicin, catechins, chlorogenic acid, curcumin, ellagic acid, lipoic acid, silymarin, sulforaphane, and terpene limonoids in your diet. See the chart "Phytonutrients: What They Do and Where to Find Them" on page 32 for more about these specific phytonutrients.

Eat a small healthy snack or meal every two to three hours to keep blood sugar levels stable. This is critical if you want to lose weight. As well, be sure to drink plenty of pure water to help flush fat out of your body.

While you learned how to clean your diet in Chapter 3, I want to emphasize that you should avoid all foods containing trans fats, MSG, artificial sweeteners, and high fructose corn syrup. These foods contribute to weight gain. And to help all your body's functions continue to work as they should, choose only organic meat, poultry, and eggs whenever possible, to avoid ingesting the hormones added to the feed of these animals.

Top 12 Fat-Fighting Foods   There are many fabulous foods that fight fat, but here are some of my favorites:

- **Green tea:** Drink between 3 and 6 cups of green tea daily to benefit from green tea's phytonutrient epigallocatechin gallate (EGCG) that speeds weight loss.

- **Leafy greens:** Spinach, spring mix, mustard greens, and other dark leafy greens are good sources of fiber and powerhouses of nutrition. Research demonstrates that their high concentration of vitamins and antioxidants helps prevent hunger while protecting you from heart disease, cancer, cataracts, and memory loss.[27]

- **Olives and olive oil:** Rich in healthy fats, olives and olive oil help to reduce cravings for junk food and keep you feeling full. Research shows that monounsaturated fats that are plentiful in these foods help reduce high blood pressure.[28]

- **Beans and legumes:** Legumes are the best source of fiber of any foods. They help to stabilize blood sugar while keeping you regular. They are also high in potassium, a critical mineral that reduces dehydration and the risk of high blood pressure and stroke. A legume, soy is particularly good for fat burning. Isoflavones found in soy foods speed the breakdown of stored fat. In one study, those who consumed high amounts of soy products shed three times more superfluous weight than those who ate no soy.[29]

- **Garlic** and **onions:** These yummy foods contain phytonutrients that break down fatty deposits in the body, while also breaking down cholesterol; killing viruses, bacteria, and fungi; and protecting against heart disease.[30]

- **Coconut oil** and **coconut milk:** Coconut contains medium chain triglycerides that reset the thyroid gland—the gland that is linked to balanced weight. Coconut oil is ideal for cooking over low to medium temperatures. Three tablespoons daily is the optimal amount.

- **Nuts:** Raw, unsalted nuts provide your body with essential fatty acids that help burn fat. Their high nutrient content also lowers the risk of heart attack by 60 percent. Research shows that consuming nuts can be as effective as cholesterol-lowering drugs to reduce high cholesterol levels, not to mention they taste better and have no nasty side effects.[31]

- **Cayenne** and **chilies:** The phytonutrient capsaicin, which gives chili peppers and cayenne their heat, lessens the risk of excess insulin in the body by speeding metabolism and lowering blood glucose (sugar) levels, before the excess insulin can result in fat stores.[32]

- **Turmeric:** A popular spice used primarily in Indian cooking, turmeric contains the highest known source of beta carotene, the antioxidant that helps protect the liver from free radical damage. Turmeric also helps your liver heal while helping your body metabolize fats by decreasing the fat storage rate in liver cells.[33]

- **Cinnamon:** Researchers at the United States Department of Agriculture showed that 1/4 to 1 teaspoon of cinnamon with food helps metabolize sugar up to 20 times better.[34] Excess sugar in the blood can lead to fat storage.

- **Flaxseed** and **flaxseed oil:** These foods attract oil-soluble toxins that are lodged in the body's fatty tissues and help escort them out.[35]

Supplementing the Diet

Supplementing your diet with a high-quality full-spectrum digestive enzyme formula that includes amylase, lipase, and protease, among other enzymes, is also beneficial. Take 1 to 3 enzyme capsules or tablets with every meal to help your body break down the carbohydrates, fats, and proteins in your food into the natural sugars, essential fatty acids, and amino acids needed for optimal healing.

It can also be helpful to supplement with one or more of the following enzymes between meals on an empty stomach: lipase, nattokinase, or superoxide dismutase (SOD), or a single product that includes some or all of these enzymes. Start with 1 capsule or tablet of your chosen enzyme(s) on an empty stomach 20 minutes before or at least 1 hour after meals, three times daily. You can gradually increase that amount to 3 capsules or tablets at a time, three times daily, or more with the guidance of a nutritional medicine practitioner who is experienced in systemic enzyme therapy.

The best natural remedies to assist in balancing weight include:

- Vitamin D3, 2000 to 4000 IU daily, to support healthy brain hormone balance
- Multivitamin and mineral, to address possible nutritional deficiencies

- Probiotics, 2 capsules at bedtime, to ensure toxins are being eliminated through the colon and not reabsorbed into the bloodstream
- Fish or flaxseed oil, 3000 mg daily of either oil, or 500 mg of DHA and 360 mg of EPA, to support healthy fat-burning processes
- L-carnitine, an amino acid, to help turn stored fat into fuel; follow package instructions, since products vary greatly
- Milk thistle, 1 teaspoon of extract twice daily for 6 weeks, to support healthy liver function

Of course, exercising at least 30 minutes daily, five days a week, is essential to weight loss. Choose both cardiovascular exercises like brisk walking, cycling, or running, along with weight lifting, which helps build muscle. When you build muscle, you actually help your body burn fat faster than if you do only cardio.

Prostate Enlargement

Located just below the bladder, the prostate gland is a chestnut-shaped gland that plays a role in the male reproductive system. While it is often considered a single gland, it is technically between 30 and 50 smaller ones with smooth muscle between them. Prostate enlargement, or benign prostatic hypertrophy, typically occurs in men over the age of 35, and the incidence increases as men age. Symptoms can include a swollen, infected prostate gland, frequent and sometimes painful need to urinate with reduced flow of urine, low back and sometimes leg pain, impotence, loss of libido, fatigue, incontinence, and painful ejaculation.

The Phytozyme Cure for Prostate Enlargement
The Diet
Most people suffering from prostate enlargement are eating more fat than their body can handle. To address these concerns, follow the Phytozyme Cure Fat Type diet outlined in Chapter 4.

Emphasize foods that contain anthocyanin, astaxanthin, beta-sitosterol, catechins, curcumin, indole-3-carbinol, isoflavones, lycopene, quercetin, resveratrol, silymarin, sulforaphane, and zeaxanthin in your diet. See the chart "Phytonutrients: What They Do and Where to Find Them" on page 32 for more about these specific phytonutrients.

Pay particular attention to eliminating food additives like colors, preservatives, and flavors, and trans fats, as well as sugar and sugar substitutes—these items will interfere with your overall health, including prostate health.

For the first several weeks of the Phytozyme Cure, drink water with the juice of one whole lemon every morning to help cleanse your body of toxic buildup. Of course, you can continue to drink the lemon water for longer if you want to. Also be sure to drink at least 8 cups of pure water daily to further eliminate toxins.

To encourage a healthy prostate, men should avoid red meat and alcohol, and reduce caffeine to no more than 1 cup of coffee or tea daily. You can drink green tea instead. Green tea's main phytonutrient, epigallocatechin gallate (EGCG), is linked to protection of the prostate against cancer.

While some people don't think it is manly to eat salads, I disagree. Salads offer such great health benefits that every man should eat at least one large green salad every day and make vegetables the focal point of meals. And if you're not crazy about vegetables, you just haven't tried the right recipes. Check out my book *The Life Force Diet* for lots of delicious nutrient-rich recipes.

Supplementing the Diet

Supplementing your diet with a high-quality full-spectrum digestive enzyme formula that includes amylase, lipase, and protease, among other enzymes, is also beneficial. Take 1 to 3 enzyme capsules or tablets with every meal to help your body break down the carbohydrates, fats, and proteins in your food into the natural sugars, essential fatty acids, and amino acids needed for optimal healing.

It can also be helpful to supplement with one or more of the following enzymes between meals on an empty stomach: bromelain, papain, serrapeptidase, superoxide dismutase (SOD), or trypsin, or a single product that includes some or all of these enzymes. Start with 1 capsule or tablet of your chosen enzyme(s) on an empty stomach 20 minutes before or at least 1 hour after meals, three times daily. You can gradually increase that amount to 3 capsules or tablets at a time, three times daily, or more with the guidance of a nutritional medicine practitioner who experienced in systemic enzyme therapy.

Supplementary turmeric is helpful to alleviate inflammation.

Zinc, which is depleted in seminal fluid, is essential for male reproductive health. Take 100 milligrams of zinc daily for the first month that you follow the Phytozyme Cure, then lower to half that dose.

As for vitamins, those who are concerned about prostate health should take a 100-milligram B-complex vitamin daily. Some of the B-complex vitamins help alleviate inflammation of the prostate, while others protect against prostate cancer. Take an additional 100 milligrams of vitamin B6. I also recommend a vitamin C supplement, because vitamin C is an excellent anti-inflammatory nutrient. Take 2000 milligrams of vitamin C every 3 hours to a total of 6000 milligrams daily for three weeks, then reduce the dose to 1500 milligrams twice daily.

I recommend two herbs in particular for men who are concerned about prostate health. Saw palmetto, an herb that acts as a tonic to the male reproductive system, is quite beneficial. Take 200 to 400 milligrams of the standardized extract daily. And pygeum africanum, sometimes referred to just as pygeum, is an herb that has proven helpful for the treatment of prostate enlargement. Take 200 to 400 milligrams of the standardized extract daily.

Of course, I cannot understate the importance of physical activity to help the body create healthy, oxygen-rich new cells. Go for a 30-minute brisk walk daily, at least three times per week, preferably five times per week, or find other activities you enjoy. Besides, participating in sports is better than watching them, anyway.

Skin Conditions (Eczema, Psoriasis)

Over 15 percent of the U.S. population is affected by either eczema or psoriasis, and drugs offer little, if any, help.

Eczema usually causes inflamed red, itchy, and dry patches of skin. Some patches may blister and weep, and eventually become crusted. It often appears in childhood and usually occurs on the face, head, elbows, knees, or the groin area. Usually caused by an allergy or food sensitivity, eczema has also been linked to immune system abnormalities like an overgrowth of the fungus *Candida albicans* or other bowel toxins, digestion difficulties, or deficiencies in essential fatty acids and other nutrients.

Psoriasis is similar in that it too frequently occurs on the scalp, knees, and elbows, but it can occur anywhere on the body. Psoriasis often shows up on the buttocks and wrists. It doesn't usually itch but may bleed if you scratch the red, swollen skin or silvery or whitish scales. It is caused by skin cells that replicate too quickly, usually around 10 times the growth rate of normal skin cells. Most scientists and doctors are mystified by what causes the skin cells to replicate at this rate. Their theories include poor diet, deficiencies in essential fatty acids and fiber, digestive difficulties, *Candida albicans* overgrowth, hormonal fluctuations, infection, stress, or poor liver function or toxic buildup.

The Phytozyme Cure for Skin Conditions

Diet

Most people suffering from eczema or psoriasis are eating more carbohydrates or fats than their body can handle. To address these concerns, follow the Phytozyme Cure Carbohydrate Type or the Phytozyme Cure Fat Type diet depending on your quiz results from Chapter 4.

Emphasize foods that contain alpha carotene, astaxanthin, beta-carotene, capsaicin, curcumin, ferulic acid, hesperetin, resveratrol, silymarin, and sulforaphane in your diet. See the chart "Phytonutrients: What They Do and Where to Find Them" on page 32 for more about these specific phytonutrients.

It is important to detoxify the bowels and liver, eliminating any possible overgrowth of *Candida albicans* or other microbes that may be infecting the body. To do that, drink plenty of water every day (usually 10 to 12 cups) to flush the bowels. Supplement with a high-quality probiotic supplement that includes *Lactobacillus acidophilus, Lactobacillus bulgaricus, Lactobacillus plantarum, Bifidobacteria,* and *Bifidobacteria bifidum.* Avoid sugars and eat only whole fruits in moderation, not fruit juices, while trying to eliminate candida. Eat protein like fish, beans, raw nuts, and seeds at every meal.

Drink more fresh vegetable juices. Your body absorbs their nutrients readily, and fresh vegetables juices are easy to digest and encourage gentle detoxification. Eat a whole foods diet consisting primarily of vegetables, fruit, nuts, seeds, and grains. However, avoid grains containing gluten—this will include foods made with whole wheat, white flour, oatmeal, spelt, and kamut—since gluten sensitivity is common in sufferers of eczema or psoriasis. I also recommend avoiding dairy products, sugar, and citrus fruits. Because alcohol often causes flare-ups, do not drink it if you suspect alcohol is implicated in your skin problems.

Supplement your diet with increased amounts of essential fatty acids, particularly omega-3s, which are found in wild salmon, flaxseed and flaxseed oil, and raw walnuts. Fish oil from a pure source provides omega-3s along with other essential fats not found in most vegetarian sources.

To improve liver function, eat more foods that support its functions, such as leafy greens, olives and olive oil (sulfite-free), beans and legumes, garlic and onions, tomatoes, raw nuts, and flaxseed and flaxseed oil. Season your food with liver-friendly spices, like cayenne pepper (not black pepper), cinnamon, and turmeric.

Supplementing the Diet

Supplementing your diet with a high-quality full-spectrum digestive enzyme formula that includes amylase, lipase, and protease, among other enzymes, is also beneficial. Take 1 to 3 enzyme capsules or tablets with every meal to help your body break down the carbohydrates, fats, and proteins in your food into the natural sugars, essential fatty acids, and amino acids needed for optimal healing.

It can also be helpful to supplement with one or more of the following enzymes between meals on an empty stomach: bromelain, lipase, papain, protease, serrapeptidase, superoxide dismutase (SOD), or trypsin, or a single product that includes some or all of these enzymes. Start with 1 capsule or tablet of your chosen enzyme(s) on an empty stomach 20 minutes before or at least 1 hour after meals, three times daily. You can gradually increase that amount to 3 capsules or tablets at a time, three times daily, or more with the guidance of a nutritional medicine practitioner experienced in systemic enzyme therapy.

In addition to being a natural and gentle colon stimulant, aloe vera juice is helpful for healing skin disorders like eczema and psoriasis. It also helps to heal the intestines, lessening chances of reinfection from candida or other microbes. Drink about 1/4 cup of aloe vera juice twice daily. Do not use if you are pregnant or lactating.

Supplement with 1000 milligrams of omega-3 fatty acids from DHA and EPA.

Eat less animal protein and supplement with a betaine hydrochloride or a hydrochloric acid supplement whenever you eat meat or fish. Take a full-spectrum digestive enzyme formula with every meal to aid digestion, lessen the chances of intestinal infection through food consumption, increase the absorption of nutrients, and lessen food sensitivities. Make sure the enzyme you take includes lipase for fat digestion, and take it alongside any essential fatty acids you consume or supplement with. Often a deficiency in essential fatty acids is the result of a lipase deficiency in the body. Supplement with the herb milk thistle containing 80 to 85 percent silymarin.

While most ointments or creams only mask the problem, many eczema and psoriasis sufferers have reported permanent relief using Cellfood Oxygen Gel, which delivers oxygen and nutrients to the skin to promote healing.

Sinus Problems (Sinusitis)

Sinusitis is an inflammation and infection of the sinuses. It is a chronic problem for most people that causes headaches, fatigue, breathing difficulty, sinus congestion, pain behind the eyes, runny nose, inflamed nasal passages, insomnia due to difficult breathing, loss of smell due to congestion, and other related symptoms. It can be linked to a fungal, viral, or bacterial infection and is often triggered by allergies.

The Phytozyme Cure for Sinus Problems
The Diet

Most people suffering from sinus infections are eating more carbohydrates, particularly sugars, than their body can handle. To address these concerns, follow the Phytozyme Cure Carbohydrate Type diet outlined in Chapter 4.

Emphasize foods that contain alpha carotene, astaxanthin, beta-carotene, capsaicin, curcumin, ferulic acid, hesperetin, proanthocyanidin, quercetin, resveratrol, tannins, and terpene limonoids in your diet. See the chart "Phytonutrients: What They Do and Where to Find Them" on page 32 for more about these specific phytonutrients. Eat mostly vegetables to get these phytonutrients and only minimal amounts of fruit.

A diet high in mucus-forming foods like dairy products, wheat, and sugar can cause the sinuses and nasal passages to become blocked, making them more vulnerable to infection. Excess salty and fried foods can also be a problem. Be sure to follow the suggestions outlined in Chapter 3 for cleaning up your diet.

The sulfur compounds found in garlic and onions assist with fighting infection of a bacterial, viral, or fungal nature (unlike pharmaceutical antibiotics, which work only on bacteria). So if you have trouble with your sinuses, incorporate more of these two foods into your daily diet.

Supplementing the Diet

Supplementing your diet with a high-quality full-spectrum digestive enzyme formula that includes amylase, lipase, and protease, among other enzymes, is also beneficial. Take 1 to 3 enzyme capsules or tablets with every meal to help your body break down the carbohydrates, fats, and proteins in your food into the natural sugars, essential fatty acids, and amino acids needed for optimal healing.

It can also be helpful to supplement with one or more of the following enzymes between meals on an empty stomach: bromelain, mucolase, papain, protease, serrapeptidase, superoxide dismutase (SOD), or trypsin, or a single product that includes some or all of these enzymes. Start with 1 capsule or tablet of your chosen enzyme(s) on an empty stomach 20 minutes before or at least 1 hour after meals, three times daily. You can gradually increase that amount to 3 capsules or tablets at a time, three times daily, or more with the guidance of a nutritional medicine practitioner experienced in systemic enzyme therapy.

The phytonutrient quercetin is particularly helpful against sinusitis, especially when it is combined with the enzyme bromelain. Take 1000 milligrams of each daily to help alleviate congestion.

Wild oregano oil is one of nature's most potent antibacterial, antiviral, and antifungal compounds. Take oregano oil drops or gel caps. Because it has a strong taste, you may prefer to take it in gel cap form. In a study reported by *ScienceDaily* magazine, oil of oregano at relatively low doses was effective against staphylococcus bacteria and was comparable to antibiotics like penicillin in its germ-killing properties. Because it is so powerful, oregano oil can also kill beneficial intestinal bacteria, so it is important to take probiotics along with any oregano oil regimen.

Researcher Paul Belaiche reported his exhaustive studies of aromatherapy oils in his three-volume work entitled *Traité de Phytothérapie et d'Aromathérapie* (Treatise on Phytotherapy and Aromatherapy). He tested the effectiveness of essential oils against specific bacteria. His findings on the effectiveness of oregano oil against many common and insidious bacteria were impressive. Belaiche found that oregano oil killed 92 percent of all staphylococcus bacteria. He also found that oregano oil eliminated 83 percent of streptococcus bacteria. Both staph and strep bacteria have been implicated in sinusitis.

The *Journal of Food Protection* cites a study by researchers at the Department of Food Science at the University of Tennessee who also report impressive findings on oregano oil's potency against bacteria. Scientists found that oregano oil exhibited the most significant antibacterial action against common germs like staphylococcus.

Because some forms of sinusitis can be caused by fungi, like the *Candida albicans* strain, following the dietary and supplement suggestions outlined under "Yeast Infections" on page 245 may be beneficial.

High doses of vitamin C can also be helpful. For acute sinusitis, take 1000 milligrams of vitamin C every hour until you reach bowel tolerance (loose stools). And then take 2000 milligrams of vitamin C every 3 to 4 hours. For chronic sinusitis, take 2000 milligrams of vitamin C every 3 to 4 hours until you reach bowel tolerance. Then take 2000 milligrams of vitamin C three times daily. You can also dissolve vitamin C crystals (make sure they are devoid of any sweeteners) into pure water and drip into your nose using a sterilized eye dropper.

Fenugreek and/or thyme herbal tea can also be helpful. Drink 3 cups daily.

Nasal washes can be valuable in treating sinusitis. You can use a basic saline solution—available in most health food stores or pharmacies—or you can mix some salt into pure water and use a neti pot (follow package directions), sold in most health food stores and many yoga studios. In addition, there is an excellent capsaicin (the main phytonutrient found in chilies) sinus spray available. A word of caution, however: While this product works marvelously, it also burns terribly for about 30 seconds or so. I find it works when almost everything else fails, but it's not for everyone.

Exercise is also important to get oxygen-rich blood circulating throughout your body, including to the sinuses, so get moving!

Sprains, Strains, and Soft Tissue Injuries

"Soft tissue" is a term commonly used to refer to the "softer" aspects of the outer body, rather than the bones and joints. Muscles, tendons, and fascia all make up soft tissues. Soft tissue injuries are commonplace and range from minor to very serious. They include sprains and strains.

Muscles are the tissues that enable us to move and stay warm. They are arranged in pairs to enable pulling and pushing types of movement. Whenever one muscle in the pair contracts, the other relaxes, and vice versa. This is the basic premise of body movement. Millions of muscle cells (also known as fibers) operate together to form muscles. Healthy muscles require a healthy diet. Well-nourished muscle cells are less likely to develop spasms or cramps that lead to pain.

If you've sustained muscle injuries, it is important to be aware of the tendency many people have to adjust their posture into a position that alleviates the pain. But this causes other muscles to overcompensate, which may create more muscular stress.

Tendons connect muscles to the bones they move. Injuries to tendons involve either a tear of some of the fibers or a complete rupture, where the tendon is torn in two. Because tendons require less blood supply than muscles to function, they take more time to heal. Chronically weakened tendons can occur anywhere, but especially around joints such as shoulders, knees, and elbows. Tendonitis is the inflammation of the tendons. Because tendons are not elastic, they're more susceptible than muscles to inflammation. The most common areas affected are the hips, knees, shoulders, heels, and elbows. To increase your tendons' resiliency, try doing a variety of activities that require a different range of motion.

The tissue that links all the components of the body together is known as fascia. It carries nerves, blood, and lymphatic vessels through it. Fascia also helps to distribute body weight during movement.

When soft tissues are injured they usually become inflamed, so it is critical to understand healthy ways to deal with inflammation.

Inflammation is a common symptom of many injuries and conditions. It is your body's healthy response to infection, tissue damage, or both. By sending increased amounts of white blood cells to the injured area, your body is better able to repair any damage. Without inflammation, injuries would not heal. Most holistic health practitioners feel that taking anti-inflammatory pharmaceuticals only masks and hence lessens the chances of proper healing.

While inflammation is the body's means of dealing with injury to soft tissues, if it remains unchecked for lengthy periods of time, it can cause serious harm to the body. However, even for short durations, inflammation can cause mobility problems and be linked with pain that is difficult to deal with.

The Phytozyme Cure for Sprains, Strains, and Soft Tissue Injuries
The Diet

People suffering from sprains, strains, or other injuries can be deficient in any or all of the enzymes needed to digest carbohydrates, fats, or proteins. If, after taking the quizzes in Chapter 4, you found that you were a Phytozyme Cure Carb, Fat, or Protein Type, follow the diet for that particular type. If you could not determine one clear type, follow the Phytozyme Cure Combination Type diet. If you frequently experience sprains, strains, or other injuries, follow the Phytozyme Cure Protein Type diet.

Emphasize foods that contain anthocyanin, astaxanthin, capsaicin, catechins, curcumin, hesperetin, and resveratrol in your diet. See the chart "Phytonutrients: What They Do and Where to Find Them" on page 32 for more about these specific phytonutrients.

Supplementing the Diet

Supplementing your diet with a high-quality full-spectrum digestive enzyme formula that includes amylase, lipase, and protease, among other enzymes, is also beneficial. Take 1 to 3 enzyme capsules or tablets with every meal to help your body break down the carbohydrates, fats, and proteins in your food into the natural sugars, essential fatty acids, and amino acids needed for optimal healing.

You can also supplement with one or more of the following enzymes between meals on an empty stomach: bromelain, nattokinase (but not immediately after surgery or if wounds are bleeding), papain, protease, serrapeptidase, or superoxide dismutase (SOD), or a single product that includes some or all of these enzymes; these enzymes can be helpful for various types of soft tissue injuries. Start with 1 capsule or tablet of your chosen enzyme(s) on an empty stomach 20 minutes before or at least 1 hour after meals, three times daily. You can gradually increase that amount to 3 capsules or tablets at a time, three times daily, or more with the guidance of a nutritional medicine practitioner who is experienced in systemic enzyme therapy.

You may recall our discussion in Chapter 3 about the long history of natural medicines. Today, the best-known pain reliever is aspirin. Aspirin's active ingredient is salicin, which converts to salicylic acid in the stomach. Chemists first synthesized salicylic acid in the nineteenth century, and the drug was given its name to reflect its herbal heritage. The herb meadowsweet was called spirea at the time. Meadowsweet, along with willow bark, contains a natural version of salicylic acid. Herbalists recommend meadowsweet or willow bark for many of the same symptoms for which doctors suggest aspirin. Herbs often have fewer side effects than pharmaceutical drugs, so that's a major benefit.

Substantial research shows that herbs like ginger, turmeric, boswellia serrata, cayenne, and guggul gum can be as effective or more effective than aspirin when used appropriately and in appropriate quantities. Also, recent findings in nutritional therapy suggest that compounds in some foods are more powerful than aspirin at alleviating pain and inflammation.

Stroke

The most important fuel for the brain is oxygen. Without it we could not live more than a few minutes. During a stroke, oxygen supply to the brain is cut off, causing brain tissues to die, often permanently. This happens because blood that carries oxygen and other nutrients to the brain is blocked or interrupted.

Stroke is the third leading cause of death in both the United States and Canada.[36,37] The vast majority of strokes are caused by arteriosclerosis—the fatty buildup inside arterial walls, which obstructs blood flow.

Too many people consider strokes an unfortunate part of aging. Strokes are usually caused, or made more likely, by lifestyle factors like poor diet, lack of exercise, smoking, and stress. The use of some medications like birth control pills, particularly in women over 35, increases the risk of stroke.

A stroke has numerous symptoms, including paralysis or numbness on one side of the face or body, confusion, dizziness, impaired speech, loss of balance, loss of consciousness, blurred vision, and a sudden severe headache.

The Phytozyme Cure for Stroke
The Diet
Most people suffering from strokes are eating more fats, particularly trans fats and animal fats, than their body can handle. To address these concerns, follow the Phytozyme Cure Fat Type diet outlined in Chapter 4.

Emphasize foods that contain anthocyanin, astaxanthin, beta-sitosterol, catechins, chlorogenic acid, curcumin, hesperetin, lipoic acid, lutein, lycopene, naringin, pectin, proanthocyanidin, resveratrol, rutin, saponins, tangeretin, and terpene limonoids in your diet. See the chart "Phytonutrients: What They Do and Where to Find Them" on page 32 for more about these specific phytonutrients.

Using Plant Nutrients to Heal and Prevent Illness

Sugar and sodium consumption can play a role in arteriosclerosis (see page 154) and therefore stroke. Excess sugar consumption increases the inflammation in artery walls, making them more susceptible to damage. Sugar is like many miniature scouring pads irritating and damaging arteries from the inside. Sodium increases blood pressure, which can increase the risk of stroke.

In a study published in the *Journal of the American Medical Association,* incremental increases of a serving of fruit or vegetables per day were linked to a decrease in stroke risk of about 6 percent.[38] So improving your diet is the first step to preventing stroke.

A long-running study conducted by Harvard University that followed 238,000 nurse participants, called The Nurses' Health Study, found a significant decrease in the risk of stroke among women who ate fish at least twice a week compared to women who ate fish only once a month.[39] In addition to eating wild fish, which is low in damaging toxins, you can supplement with fish oil that contains 100 milligrams of EPA and 500 milligrams of DHA daily to help reduce arterial inflammation while lowering cholesterol and triglyceride levels.

Supplementing the Diet

Supplementing your diet with a high-quality full-spectrum digestive enzyme formula that includes amylase, lipase, and protease, among other enzymes, is also beneficial. Take 1 to 3 enzyme capsules or tablets with every meal to help your body break down the carbohydrates, fats, and proteins in your food into the natural sugars, essential fatty acids, and amino acids needed for optimal healing.

It can also be helpful to supplement with one or more of the following enzymes between meals on an empty stomach: bromelain, catalase, lipase, papain, protease, serrapeptidase, superoxide dismutase (SOD), or trypsin, or a single product that includes some or all of these enzymes. Start with 1 capsule or tablet of your chosen enzyme(s) on an empty stomach 20 minutes before or at least 1 hour after meals, three times daily. You can gradually increase that amount to 3 capsules or tablets at a time, three times daily, or more with the guidance of a nutritional medicine practitioner who is experienced in systemic enzyme therapy.

. Take a high-potency, high-quality multivitamin and mineral daily to obtain a variety of antioxidants and important minerals proven to reduce stroke risk and prevent nutritional deficiencies.

Take 400 IU of mixed tocopherols found in a vitamin E supplement to help thin blood and prevent cholesterol from oxidizing in the blood vessels.

Ginkgo biloba is a powerful antioxidant that also has blood-thinning properties. Take between 60 and 120 milligrams twice daily of a product containing 24 percent glycosides and 6 percent terpene lactones for maximum benefit.

In some animal studies, coenzyme Q10 (CoQ10) has prevented neurological damage from stroke.[40] It is essential to manufacturing energy in all cells, including neurons. Take 200 milligrams daily.

NADH (nicotinamide adenine dinucleotide) has shown an ability to revitalize the metabolism of damaged neurons, making it suitable for inclusion in a natural medicine program for stroke. Take 5 milligrams twice daily.

Green tea *(Camellia sinensis)*, in addition to its ability to support important probiotics needed for brain health, is a rich source of antioxidants that lessen free radical damage and promote detoxification. Choose a product that is standardized to 80 to 90 percent polyphenols and 35 to 55 percent epigallocatechin gallate (EGCG), both important natural compounds with brain health–promoting qualities. Drinking green tea can be beneficial for stroke sufferers, but supplementing with a standardized extract of green tea's effective compounds will have even greater therapeutic effects.

Research also shows that policosanol reduces total and LDL cholesterol while increasing the good HDL cholesterol levels. Policosanol is a natural compound extracted from sugarcane wax, beeswax, or rice bran wax. Studies show policosanol is equally effective as pharmaceutical medications to lower cholesterol levels. However, it is superior to drugs in its ability to raise HDL (good) cholesterol. Take 10 to 20 milligrams every evening.

Vinpocetine, an extract from the periwinkle plant, shows tremendous promise in stroke rehabilitation. Take 5 milligrams twice daily as a therapeutic dose.

To reduce homocysteine levels, which are typically high in stroke patients, supplement with folate and vitamins B6 and B12, all of which are helpful to reduce this harmful compound. Take 800 micrograms of folate, 100 milligrams of vitamin B6, and 200 micrograms of vitamin B12.

Acetyl-L-carnitine transports fuel into the cells for energy production and helps eliminate cellular waste products, both of which are important to stroke recovery. Take 400 milligrams daily for stroke recovery.

Phosphatidylserine (PS) plays an important role in increasing energy production at the cellular level, while improving cell-to-cell communication, making it an important nutrient in the natural treatment of stroke. Take 100 milligrams daily. (To read more about PS, refer to the section on ADHD/ADD on page 148.)

Yeast Infections

Vaginal yeast infections, also called vaginitis, are the result of a fungal overgrowth in the vaginal area. A yeast infection can be caused by bacteria, as is the case with gonorrhea, protozoans (usually trichomonas), yeast, and fungus. The specific type of fungus most commonly responsible for yeast infections is *Candida albicans*. I discussed *Candida albicans* as it pertained to intestinal overgrowth in Chapter 3. Much of that information is relevant to vaginal candida overgrowth as well. Usually, a woman with vaginitis also has an intestinal candida overgrowth that needs to be addressed.

The Phytozyme Cure for Yeast Infections
The Diet

Most people suffering from yeast infections are eating more protein or sugars than their body can handle. To address these concerns, follow the Phytozyme Cure Protein Type or the Phytozyme Cure Carbohydrate Type diet outlined in Chapter 4.

Emphasize foods that contain alpha carotene, anthocyanin, beta-carotene, catechins, curcumin, ferulic acid, hesperetin, pectin, resveratrol, and sulforaphane in your diet. See the chart "Phytonutrients: What They Do and Where to Find Them" on page 32 for more about these specific phytonutrients.

Be sure to follow the dietary suggestions for the Phytozyme Cure as outlined in Chapter 3. Pay particular attention to avoiding sugar and sugar substitutes until the infection is gone. That means you should eat only minimal fruit and eliminate alcohol completely during this time. Once the infection appears to be gone, follow a low-sugar diet to prevent future infections. While certain drugs and natural approaches can help with yeast infections, the reality is that without a long-term change in diet and lifestyle, the infections are likely to keep coming back.

Supplementing the Diet

Supplementing your diet with a high-quality full-spectrum digestive enzyme formula that includes amylase, lipase, and protease, among other enzymes, is also beneficial. Take 1 to 3 enzyme capsules or tablets with every meal to help your body break down the carbohydrates, fats, and proteins in your food into the natural sugars, essential fatty acids, and amino acids needed for optimal healing.

It can also be helpful to supplement with one or more of the following enzymes between meals on an empty stomach: cellulose, chymotrypsin, papain, protease, serrapeptidase, superoxide dismutase (SOD), or trypsin, or a single product that includes some or all of these enzymes. Start with 1 capsule or tablet of your chosen enzyme(s) on an empty stomach 20 minutes before or at least 1 hour after meals, three times daily. You can gradually increase that amount to 3 capsules or tablets at a time, three times daily, or more with the guidance of a nutritional medicine practitioner who is experienced in systemic enzyme therapy.

Supplement with wild oregano oil in drop or gel cap form. Because it has a strong taste, I find that most people prefer to take gel caps. Researcher Paul Belaiche reported his exhaustive studies of aromatherapy oils in his three-volume work entitled *Traité de Phytothérapie et d'Aromathérapie* (Treatise on Phytotherapy and Aromatherapy). He tested the effectiveness of essential oils against specific bacteria. His findings on the effectiveness of oregano oil against many common and insidious bacteria were impressive. He found that oregano oil killed 78 percent of candida bacteria, commonly linked with intestinal or systemic candida infections. Because it is so powerful, oregano oil can also kill beneficial intestinal bacteria, so it is important to take probiotics along with any oregano oil regimen—be sure you are taking 2 capsules of a high-quality probiotic supplement nightly on an empty stomach. Also, be sure to take oregano oil and probiotics a few hours apart.

Endnotes

Chapter 1

1. Classifications of phytonutrients in this book were adapted from John W. Erdman Jr. et al., "Flavonoids and Heart Health: Proceedings of the ILSI North America Flavonoids Workshop, May 31-June 1, 2005, Washington, DC." *Journal of Nutrition,* http://ddr.nal.usda.gov/dspace/bitstream/10113/12494/1/IND43882671.pdf, accessed January 12, 2010.

2. Lester Packer and Carol Colman, *The Antioxidant Miracle* (New York: John Wiley and Sons, 1999), 134.

3. AOL Health, "Phytonutrients: Prevention in a Plant," http://body.aol.com/medical-myths/phytonutrients-prevention-in-a-plant, accessed January 10, 2010.

4. Ibid.

5. John R. Smythies, *Every Person's Guide to Antioxidants* (Piscataway, NJ: Rutgers University Press, 1998), 45.

6. Brenda Kearns, "Superfood discovery," *First for Women,* June 9, 2008: 30-33.

7. Barbara L. Minton. "Astaxanthin is age and disease defying miracle micronutrient from microalgae," *Natural News,* http://www.naturalnews.com/026309_astaxanthin_cancer_disease.html, accessed January 14, 2010.

8. *On free radical damage to the liver:* G.D. Curek et al., "Effect of astaxanthin on hepatocellular injury following ischemia/reperfusion," Toxicology, November 10, 2009, http://www.ncbi.nlm.nih.gov/pubmed/19990500?itool=EntrezSystem2.PEntrez.Pubmed.Pubmed_ResultsPanel.Pubmed_RVDocSum&ordinalpos=10, accessed January 14, 2010. *On liver cancer:* D.N. Tripathi and G.B. Jena, "Astaxanthin intervention ameliorates cyclophosphamide-induced oxidative stress, DNA damage and early hepatocarcinogenesis in rat: Role of Nrf2, p53, p38 and phase-II enzymes," Mutation Research, December 28, 2009, http://www.ncbi.nlm.nih.gov/pubmed/20038455?itool=EntrezSystem2.PEntrez.Pubmed.Pubmed_ResultsPanel.Pubmed_RVDocSum&ordinalpos=4, accessed January 14, 2010. *On colon cancer:* P. Nagendraprabhu and G. Sudhandiran, "Astaxanthin inhibits tumor invasion by decreasing extracellular matrix production and induces apoptosis in experimental rat colon carcinogenesis by modulating the expressions of ERK-2, NFkB and COX-2," Investigational New Drugs, October 30, 2009, http://www.ncbi.nlm.nih.gov/pubmed/19876598?itool=EntrezSystem2.PEntrez.Pubmed.Pubmed_ResultsPanel.Pubmed_RVDocSum&ordinalpos=13, accessed January 14, 2010.

9. Mike Adams, "Astaxanthin sources revealed: Super antioxidant eases arthritis pain, joint pain, sore muscles and protects against heart disease," Natural News, http://www.naturalnews.com/002156.html, accessed March 30, 2010.

10. Daniel Q. Haney and Warren King, "Beta Carotene May Cause, Not Prevent, Cancer," http://community.seattletimes.nwsource.com/archive/?date=19940413 &slug=1905322, accessed January 14, 2010.

11. Lester Packer and Carol Colman, *The Antioxidant Miracle* (New York: John Wiley and Sons, 1999), 137.

12. Ibid., 138.

13. "What Is Beta-Sitosterol?" Phytochemicals. http://www.phytochemicals.info/ phytochemicals/beta-sitosterol.php, accessed March 30, 2010.

14. "What Is Capsaicin?" Phytochemicals.info, http://www.phytochemicals.info/ phytochemicals/capsaicin.php, accessed March 30, 2010.

15. Brenda Kearns, "Superfood discovery," *First for Women,* June 9, 2008: 30-33.

16. Lester Packer and Carol Colman, *The Antioxidant Miracle* (New York: John Wiley and Sons, 1999), 139.

17. Michael Colgan, "Save Your Brain," 2007. Vista, www.vistamagonline.com/ articles.

18. Michelle Schoffro Cook, *Healing Injuries the Natural Way* (Toronto: Your Health Press, 2004).

19. "What Is Ferulic Acid?" Phytochemicals.info, http://www.phytochemicals.info/ phytochemicals/ferulic-acid.php, accessed March 30, 2010.

20. Ibid.

21. "Hesperidin," Phytochemicals.info, http://www.phytochemicals.info/phy tochemicals/hesperidin.php, accessed January 21, 2010.

22. Ibid.

23. "What Is Indole-3-Carbinol?" Phytochemicals.info, http://www.phytochemi cals.info/phytochemicals/indole-3-carbinol.php, accessed March 30, 2010.

24. "Genistein," Phytochemicals.info, http://www.phytochemicals.info/phy tochemicals/genistein.php, accessed January 20, 2010.

25. Ibid.

26. Brenda Kearns, "Superfood discovery," *First for Women,* June 9, 2008: 30-33.

27. Joseph Mercola, "Antioxidant Lutein Decreases Heart Disease," http://articles .mercola.com/sites/articles/archive/2001/07/04/lutein.aspx, accessed January 14, 2010.

28. "Atherosclerosis," The World's Healthiest Foods, George Mateljan Foundation, http://whfoods.org/genpage.php?tname=disease&dbid=4#summary, accessed January 14, 2010.

29. John R. Smythies, *Every Person's Guide to Antioxidants* (Piscataway, NJ: Rutgers University Press, 1998), 45.

30. **On prostate cancer:** Joseph Mercola, "Synthetic Lycopene Slows Prostate Cancer," http://blogs.mercola.com/sites/vitalvotes/archive/2004/09/30/syn thetic-lycopene-slows-prostate-cancer.aspx, accessed January 14, 2010. **On atherosclerosis:** Joseph Mercola, "Lycopene May Help Prevent Atherosclerosis,"

http://articles.mercola.com/sites/articles/archive/2000/12/31/lycopene-heart.
aspx, accessed January 14, 2010. *On asthma:* Joseph Mercola, "Lycopene
May Protect Against Asthma," http://articles.mercola.com/sites/articles/
archive/2001/01/07/lycopene-asthma.aspx, accessed January 14, 2010.

31. R.B. van Breemen and N. Pajkovic, "Multitargeted therapy of cancer by lycopene," *Cancer Letters*, October 8, 2008, http://www.ncbi.nlm.nih.gov/pubm
ed/18585855?ordinalpos=1&itool=EntrezSystem2.PEntrez.Pubmed.Pubmed_
ResultsPanel.Pubmed_MultiItemSupl.Pubmed_TitleSearch&linkpos=2&log$
=pmtitlesearch4, accessed January 15, 2010.

32. G. Banhegyi, "Lycopene—a natural antioxidant," *Orvosi Hetilap*, July 31, 2005,
http://www.ncbi.nlm.nih.gov/pubmed/16158610?ordinalpos=1&itool=EntrezSyst
em2.PEntrez.Pubmed.Pubmed_ResultsPanel.Pubmed_SingleItemSupl.Pubmed_
Discovery_RA&linkpos=4&log$=relatedreviews&logdbfrom=pubmed, accessed
January 15, 2010.

33. S. Agarwal and A.V. Rao, "Tomato lycopene and its role in human health and
chronic diseases," *Canadian Medical Association Journal*, September 19, 2000,
http://www.ncbi.nlm.nih.gov/pubmed/11022591?ordinalpos=1&itool=EntrezSyst
em2.PEntrez.Pubmed.Pubmed_ResultsPanel.Pubmed_SingleItemSupl.Pubmed_
Discovery_RA&linkpos=2&log$=relatedreviews&logdbfrom=pubmed, accessed
January 15, 2010.

34. H.N. Saada et al., "Lycopene protects the structure of the small intestines,"
Phytotherapy Research, December 29, 2009, http://www.ncbi.nlm.nih.gov/pub
med/20041432?itool=EntrezSystem2.PEntrez.Pubmed.Pubmed_ResultsPanel
.Pubmed_RVDocSum&ordinalpos=5, accessed January 15, 2010.

35. "Naringin," Phytochemicals.info, http://www.phytochemicals.info/phytochem
icals/naringin.php, accessed January 21, 2010.

36. Ibid.

37. V. Gaur, "Protective effect of naringin against ischemic reperfusion cerebral
injury: Possible neurobehavioral, biochemical and cellular alterations in rat
brain," http://www.ncbi.nlm.nih.gov/pubmed/19577560?ordinalpos=1&itool=
EntrezSystem2.PEntrez.Pubmed.Pubmed_ResultsPanel.Pubmed_SingleItem
Supl.Pubmed_Discovery_RA&linkpos=3&log$=relatedarticles&logdbfrom=
pubmed, accessed January 21, 2010.

38. M.Y. Kotimchenko and E.A. Kolenchenko, "Efficiency of low-esterified pectin
in toxic damage to the liver inflicted by lead treatment," *Bulletin of Experimental
Biology and Medicine,* July 2007, http://www.ncbi.nlm.nih.gov/pubmed/182567
53?ordinalpos=1&itool=EntrezSystem2.PEntrez.Pubmed.Pubmed_ResultsPanel
.Pubmed_SingleItemSupl.Pubmed_Discovery_RA&linkpos=2&log$=relateda
rticles&logdbfrom=pubmed, accessed January 20, 2010.

39. Ben Best, "Phytochemicals as Nutraceuticals," http://www.benbest.com/nutr
ceut/phytochemicals.html, accessed January 13, 2010.

40. J. Robert Hatherill, *The BrainGate: The Little-Known Doorway That Lets Nutrients In and Keeps Toxic Agents Out* (Washington, DC: Lifeline Press, 2003), 89.

41. "What Is Proanthocyanidin?" Phytochemicals.info, http://www.phytochemi cals.info/phytochemicals/proanthocyanidins.php, accessed March 30, 2010.

42. "Quercetin," Phytochemicals.info, http://www.phytochemicals.info/phy tochemicals/quercetin.php, accessed January 21, 2010.

43. "Resveratrol," Phytochemicals.info, http://www.phytochemicals.info/phy tochemicals/resveratrol.php, accessed January 20, 2010.

44. *On preventing your intestines from absorbing it:* Y. Matsui et al. "Quantita tive analysis of saponins in a tea-leaf extract and their anti-hypercholesterolemic activity," *Bioscience, Biotechnology, and Biochemistry*, July 2009. http://www .ncbi.nlm.nih.gov/pubmed/19584556?itool=EntrezSystem2.PEntrez.Pubmed .Pubmed_ResultsPanel.Pubmed_RVDocSum&ordinalpos=10, accessed January 15, 2010. *On colon cancer:* Ben Best, "Phytochemicals as Nutraceuticals," http:// www.benbest.com/nutrceut/phytochemicals.html, accessed January 13, 2010.

45. Andrea Marshall, "Milk Thistle Benefits Are Due to Silymarin," http://ezineart icles.com/?Milk-Thistle-Benefits-Are-Due-to-Silymarin&id=2186050, accessed March 29, 2010.

46. "What Is Sulforaphane?" Phytochemicals.info, http://www.phytochemicals .info/phytochemicals/sulforaphane.php, accessed March 30, 2010.

47. Brenda Kearns, "Superfood discovery," *First for Women*, June 9, 2008: 30-33.

48. "What Is Tangeretin?" Phytochemicals.info, http://www.phytochemicals.info/ phytochemicals/tangeretin.php, accessed March 29, 2010.

49. Ibid.

50. Ibid.

51. G.D. Manners, "Citrus limonoids: Analysis, bioactivity, and biomedical pros pects," *Journal of Agriculture and Food Chemistry*, October 17, 2007, http://www .ncbi.nlm.nih.gov/pubmed/17892257?itool=EntrezSystem2.PEntrez.Pubmed .Pubmed_ResultsPanel.Pubmed_RVDocSum&ordinalpos=4, accessed January 14, 2010.

52. Joseph Mercola, "The Two Superfoods That Stop Blindness," http://articles .mercola.com/sites/articles/archive/2007/09/25/the-two-superfoods-that-stop- blindness.aspx, accessed January 14, 2010.

53. Joseph Mercola, "Why You Want to Be Sure and Take Antioxidants When You Fly," http://blogs.mercola.com/sites/vitalvotes/archive/2009/10/15/why-you-want- to-be-sure-and-take-antioxidants-when-you-fly.aspx, accessed January 14, 2010.

Chapter 2

1. Willcox and Matatov, "The enzyme cure," *First for Women,* July 30, 2007: 30-33.

2. Ibid.

3. Edward Howell, *Enzyme Nutrition* (Wayne, NJ: Avery, 1985).

4. Hiromi Shinya, *The Enzyme Factor* (San Francisco: Council Oak Books, 2005), 34.

5. Tom Bohager, *Everything You Need to Know About Enzymes* (Austin: Greenleaf Book Group Press, 2008), 14.

6. Ibid., 15.

7. Anthony J. Cichoke, *Enzymes & Enzyme Therapy* (Los Angeles: Keats Publishing, 2000), 163.

8. "Worldwide AIDS & HIV Statistics," AVERT, http://www.avert.org/world stats.htm.

9. Anthony J. Cichoke, *Enzymes & Enzyme Therapy* (Los Angeles: Keats Publishing, 2000), 163.

10. Humbert Santillo, *Food Enzymes: The Missing Link to Radiant Health* (Prescott, AZ: Hohm Press, 1993), 36.

11. Michael Loes and David Steinman, *The Aspirin Alternative: The Natural Way to Overcome Chronic Pain, Reduce Inflammation, and Enhance the Healing Response* (Topanga, CA: Freedom Press, 1999), 62.

12. Ibid., 66.

13. Ibid.

14. F. Singer and H. Obleitner, "Drug therapy of activated arthrosis: On the effectiveness of an enzyme mixture versus diclofenac," *Wien Med Wochenschr* 146(3): 55-58, http://www.ncbi.nlm.nih.gov/pubmed/8867274, accessed April 13, 2010.

15. A.B. Volosianko, "The dynamics of the humoral immunity indices and of the beta 2-microglobulin level in children with chronic hepatitis," *Lik Sprava*, 2000 March (2): 67-69, http://www.ncbi.nlm.nih.gov/pubmed/10862480, accessed April 13, 2010.

16. Anthony J. Cichoke, *Enzymes & Enzyme Therapy* (Los Angeles: Keats Publishing, 2000), 93-95; Anthony J. Cichoke, *The Complete Book of Enzyme Therapy* (Garden City Park, NY: Avery, 1999), 45-54.

17. Lita Lee and Lisa Turner, *The Enzyme Cure: How Plant Enzymes Can Help You Relieve 36 Health Problems* (Tiburon, CA: Future Medicine Publishing, 1998), 164.

18. Anthony J. Cichoke, *Enzymes & Enzyme Therapy* (Los Angeles: Keats Publishing, 2000), 94.

19. J. Beuth, "Proteolytic enzyme therapy in evidence-based complementary oncology: Fact or fiction?" *Integrative Cancer Therapies* 7(4): 311-16, http://www.ncbi.nlm.nih.gov/pubmed/19116226, accessed April 13, 2010.

20. E. Zavadova et al., "Stimulation of reactive oxygen species production and cytotoxicity in human neutrophils in vitro and after oral administration of a polyenzyme preparation," *Cancer Biotherapy* 10(2): 147-52, http://www.ncbi.nlm.nih.gov/pubmed/7663574, accessed April 13, 2010.

21. A. Sakalova et al., "The favorable effect of hydrolytic enzymes in the treatment of immunocytomas and plasmacytomas," *Vnitr Lek* 38(9): 921-29, http://www.ncbi.nlm.nih.gov/pubmed/1481392, accessed April 13, 2010.

22. J. Adamek et al., "Enzyme therapy in the treatment of lymphedema in the arm after breast carcinoma surgery," *Rozhl Chir* 76(4): 203-4, http://www.ncbi.nlm .nih.gov/pubmed/9265253, accessed April 13, 2010.

23. H.O. Hubarieva et al., "Systemic enzymotherapy as a method of prophylaxis of postradiation complications in oncological patients," *Lik Sprava,* October-December 2000 (7-8): 94-100, http://www.ncbi.nlm.nih.gov/pubmed/16786662, accessed April 13, 2010.

24. K. Bhui et al., "Bromelain inhibits COX-2 expression by blocking the activation of MAPK regulated NF-kappa B against skin tumor-initiation triggering mitochondrial death pathway," *Cancer Letters* 282(2): 167-76, http://www.ncbi .nlm.nih.gov/pubmed/19339108, accessed April 13, 2010.

25. M. Wald, "Exogenous proteases confer a significant chemopreventive effect in experimental tumor models," *Integrative Cancer Therapies* 7(4): 295-310, http:// www.ncbi.nlm.nih.gov/sites/entrez, accessed April 13, 2010.

26. Ibid.

27. R. Kleef et al., "Selective modulation of cell adhesion molecules on lymphocytes by bromelain protease 5," *Pathobiology* 64(6): 339-46, http://www.ncbi.nlm.nih .gov/pubmed/9159029, accessed April 13, 2010.

28. A.V. Everitt et al., "Life extension by calorie restriction in humans." Annals of the New York Academy of Sciences. 2007 Oct; 1114:428-33. Epub 2007 Aug 23.

29. Tom Bohager, *Everything You Need to Know About Enzymes* (Austin: Greenleaf Book Group Press, 2008).

30. Ellen W. Cutler with Jeremy E. Kaslow, *MicroMiracles: Discover the Healing Power of Enzymes* (Rodale, 2005), 295-319.

31. National Enzyme Company and TNO Nutrition and Food Research, "The first quantitative evidence proving the efficacy of supplemental enzymes," http:// www.nationalenzyme.com/PDF-NEWS/NEC_TNO_Efficacy_Study.pdf, accessed February 8, 2010.

32. Tom Bohager, *Everything You Need to Know About Enzymes* (Austin: Greenleaf Book Group Press, 2008), 54-57.

33. Anthony J. Cichoke, *The Complete Book of Enzyme Therapy* (Garden City Park, NY: Avery, 1999), 45-54.

34. Anthony J. Cichoke, *Enzymes & Enzyme Therapy* (Los Angeles: Keats Publishing, 2000).

Chapter 3

1. Lynne Melcombe, *Health Hazards of White Sugar* (Vancouver: Alive Books, 2001).

2. Nancy Appleton, *Lick the Sugar Habit* (New York: Avery, 1996).

3. Russell L. Blaylock, *Excitotoxins: The Taste That Kills* (Santa Fe: Health Press NA, 1997), 42.

4. Ibid., 255-56.

5. Ibid., 38.

6. Ibid., 75.

7. Ibid., 125.

8. E. Liu et al., "Predicted 25-hydroxyvitamin D score and incident type 2 diabetes in the Framingham Offspring Study," *Am J Clin Nutr.* 2010 Jun;91(6):1627-33. Epub 2010 Apr 14 http://www.ncbi.nlm.nih.gov/pubmed/20392893, accessed March 25, 2010.

9. Joseph Mercola, "Vitamin D Deficiency Is Why You Get the Flu!" http://articles.mercola.com/sites/articles/archive/2010/03/25/vitamin-d-deficiency-is-why-you-get-flu.aspx, accessed April 19, 2010.

10. Ibid.

Chapter 4

1. Lita Lee, Lisa Turner, et al., *The Enzyme Cure* (Tiburon, CA: Future Medicine Publishing, 1998), 38; Apex Energetics Notes; Ellen W. Cutler with Jeremy E. Kaslow, *Micro Miracles* (Emmaus, PA: Rodale, 2005), 53-54.

2. Dietary suggestions are based on information in Ellen W. Cutler with Jeremy E. Kaslow, *Micro Miracles* (Emmaus, PA: Rodale, 2005).

Part Two

1. James Balch and Mark Stengler, *Prescription for Natural Cures* (Hoboken, NJ: John Wiley and Sons, 2004), 68.

2. R.J. Prinz et al., "Dietary correlates of hyperactive behaviour in children," *Journal of Consulting and Clinical Psychology* 48: 760-69.

3. L. Langseth and J. Dowd, "Glucose tolerance and hyperkinesis," *Food and Cosmetics Toxicology* 16: 129.

4. Patrick Holford, *The New Optimum Nutrition Bible* (Toronto: Crossing Press, 2004), 358.

5. James Balch and Mark Stengler, *Prescription for Natural Cures* (Hoboken, NJ: John Wiley and Sons, 2004), 71.

6. Michael Loes and David Steinman, *The Aspirin Alternative* (Topanga, CA: Freedom Press, 2001), 84.

7. Brenda Kearns, "Eat this to prevent breast cancer!" *Woman's World*, November 23, 2009: 16.

8. Ibid.

9. Linda Page, *Linda Page's Healthy Healing: A Guide to Self-Healing for Everyone,* 12th ed. (Healthy Healing, 2006), 346.

10. Linda Page, *Linda Page's Healthy Healing: A Guide to Self-Healing for Everyone,* 12th ed. (Healthy Healing, 2006), 400.

11. Patrick Holford, *The New Optimum Nutrition Bible* (Toronto: Crossing Press, 2004), 655.

12. Ibid., 142-43.

13. Ibid., 139.

14. Ibid., 140.

15. Ibid.

16. Ibid.

17. Ibid., 141.

18. Ibid., 142.

19. Ibid., 143-44.

20. Ibid., 138.

21. Ibid.

22. Linda Page, *Linda Page's Healthy Healing: A Guide to Self-Healing for Everyone*, 12th ed. (Healthy Healing, 2006), 489.

23. "Anti-inflammatory drugs dramatically reduce Parkinson's risk," *Archive of Neurology*, 2003 (60): 1059-64.

24. Stephanie Beling, *Power Foods* (New York: HarperCollins, 1997), 178.

25. Ibid.

26. Ibid.

27. "Fat-burning foods," *Woman's World*, April 27, 2004: 18-21.

28. Ibid.

29. Ibid.

30. Ibid.

31. Ibid.

32. Ann Louise Gittleman, *The Fat Flush Plan* (New York: McGraw-Hill, 2002), 35.

33. Ibid., 19.

34. Ibid., 35.

35. Ibid., 42.

36. Patrick Casanova. "Multiple Chemical Sensitivity: A Literary Critique," Environmental Illness Resource, http://www.ei-resource.org/Articles/mcs-art04.asp, accessed July 2006.

37. Heart and Stroke Foundation, "Statistics," http://www.heartandstroke.com/site/c.ikIQLcMWJtE/b.3483991/k.34A8/Statistics.htm, accessed May 18, 2010.

38. KJ Joshipura et al. "Fruit and vegetable intake in relation to risk of ischemic stroke" JAMA, 1999 (13): 1233-9.

39. James Balch and Mark Stengler, *Prescription for Natural Cures* (Hoboken, NJ: John Wiley and Sons, 2004), 488.

40. Clifford Shults. "Coenzyme Q10 slows progression of Parkinson's," *Archives of Neurology*, 2002 (59): 1541-50.

Index